Losing the Weight
Loving Yourself, Living Your Best Life, and Losing the Darn Weight

By:
Summerlin Conner

For a more immersive experience, you may enjoy the companion journal/planner to this book (available on Amazon):
A Companion Journal For Losing The Weight: A Year's Worth of Self-Care, Self-Love, and Weight Loss

Also by *Summerlin Conner*:

The Three of Us: A Brutally Honest, Often Hilarious, and Sometimes Heartbreaking Memoir of One Mom's Adventures in Single Parenting

The Single Mom's Little Guide to Building a Big Life

For Mom and Dad, my angels looking over me

If you want to fly, give up everything that's weighing you down.

-Buddha

Table of Contents

Introduction

One day I was sitting on my couch watching a movie. In one scene, a woman walks into a crowded living room where a festive party is going on. She's a large woman. She's dressed nicely and looks pretty, but she's very overweight. She has a giant smile on her face and quickly and easily makes her rounds in the room saying hello to her friends. She looks genuinely happy. The rest of the story doesn't matter. Just that one scene. Why does only that one scene matter? Because that's the moment when something clicked for me.

While I watched this party scene unfolding, my thoughts were of shock and horror. *How on Earth does she just breeze on into that darn party like nobody's business? Why isn't she looking nervous and immediately heading for the corner? Doesn't she know she's fat? She must have lost her dang mind! Maybe she seriously doesn't even know she's fat? My gosh, I wish I could do that. She actually looks freaking happy! What on Earth!?*

Now, before you go thinking that I am fat shaming someone, I swear to you that I am 100% not. I was thirty pounds overweight myself when this happened. The thing is, I genuinely was perplexed at how a large woman could even remotely be happy. I was genuinely flustered by the thought of breezing into a party without trying to immediately hide in the corner. I honestly couldn't understand how she could have even a morsel of pride. I couldn't wrap my mind around this combination of being overweight and happy. In my mind, the two just didn't go together. I couldn't understand how she could love her larger body because I had NEVER been able to love mine. For my entire life, I judged myself based on my body size. When I was fat, I was unlovable. When I was thin, I was lovable. End of story.

I have tried every diet there is. I have starved, binged, and everything in between. My body has been all shapes and all sizes. I have been underweight and overweight. I ate way too much and I ate way too little. One thing, though, has remained constant for me. I have always had a dysfunctional relationship with food.

Since my twenties, I have been on a roller coaster ride of ballooning up and shrinking down over and over. There were periods where my body was trim and toned and in good shape. And periods where my body was obese and sickly and stagnant.

The most constant element throughout all this time is that I have always been thinking about food. I have been obsessed with food. Thinking about when I will eat next. Thinking about what I will eat. Planning new diets. Brainstorming new ways to control my eating. Kicking myself for binging. Praising myself for eating "right." Figuring out how to sneak away and stuff myself with donuts. Thinking about how not to think about food. Obsessing over trying to figure out how not to be obsessed any more. Phew.

Looking back, I can somewhat see a correlation between my body size and particular stages of my life. For instance, after getting divorced and becoming a single parent, I gained about thirty pounds within just a year or two. I had no time for exercise and healthy eating. Okay, that makes sense. And when my kids were in elementary school and my life was pretty "together," I was mostly trim and toned. That makes sense also. Regardless, in both instances I was still obsessing about food the ENTIRE time.

If you have ever in your life been in this kind of battle with food and eating, then you know what kind of torture this is. It is absolutely nightmarish. The highs and the lows. The excitement over starting a new diet and then the horrendous despair and crushing defeat when you fail at it. Again.

I can't tell you how many times I have gotten all worked up and excited about a new diet. Starting a new diet feels like the greatest thing in the world. There is so much hope for the future and a better life ahead. And you are absolutely certain that THIS TIME it will work. You get all the food together and learn everything you can about this diet. You have so much excitement you can barely stand it. And you are convinced that this diet is the perfect one for you and *what had you been thinking with all those other ones?* You spend your time daydreaming about your new body and all the amazing clothes you will wear and how INCREDIBLE it will feel to put that cute little bathing suit on and head to the beach. You just know that in a few short months your whole life will be so much better with your new body! You will go out more, feel more confident, look incredible, and everything will be just perfect.

And then you start the diet. A few days go by and things are going really well! So far, this diet isn't so bad at all. You get on the scale and you have lost a pound or two!! Yes!! You think to yourself, *This is it! I am losing the weight and my life is changing and I am doing this!* A few more days go by, maybe a week. Slowly but surely you start to get a little tired and come back down to Earth from the initial high of starting the diet. Real life starts creeping back in. The kids are hungry, work is exhausting, the dog is barking, and so on and so on. And then, like clockwork, the cravings start sneaking up on you. *You know, today was really crappy and that chocolate chip cookie looks so freaking good and soothing and probably just one wouldn't hurt, right?*

For the first few cravings you fight through it with all your might and don't cave in. But somewhere along the line, the cravings are stronger than you can take. Maybe you had a really crappy day. Maybe you are exhausted and there was major drama at work today. Maybe the kids have been fighting nonstop and your nerves are fried. Whatever the reason, food sounds so comforting and irresistible. So you cave.

Those first few bites are like heaven. Nothing has ever tasted better. It feels like you have been in jail and then set free. It feels like your body has been tortured and deprived and now it is being cared for and nourished. And your mood immediately changes. You feel SO GOOD. It's like an instant high with those first few bites. Cake, donuts, chips, pizza, ice cream, whatever; it doesn't matter. It's whatever you were craving that is now like Heaven to your mouth and your mood.

At first, there is no guilt. You are feeling so freaking good and honestly believe that you are doing the right thing because it feels so good. It feels so right. So you keep eating. And eating. Next thing you know you have eaten the whole pint of ice cream or the whole sleeve of Girl Scout cookies. But you can't stop. You think to yourself, *Tomorrow I will have to go back on the diet so I have to get as much as I can now because who knows when I will get to eat this yummy stuff again?* So you keep right on eating. You start getting really full but you can't stop. IT TASTES SO GOOD!! And you have been missing it so much. It's like a long-lost friend who you haven't been able to see in forever and you don't know when you will see them again. You have to take in as much as you possibly can right now. So you have a few more bites.

And then you start feeling really sick. It still tastes good, but you are starting to feel slightly nauseated. And the initial high you felt is slowly dying off. You are starting to come back down to Earth and reality. But there is still a little bit of cake left and it still looks really good and seriously it might be forever before you get to eat something like this again. So just a few more bites. And then a few more. Okay, now you are really not feeling so well. Your stomach is bloated and nauseous. Your high has completely crashed down. Now you are kicking yourself. *Oh my God, what did I just do? What is WRONG with me?? I am so fat and so disgusting. I cannot believe what an absolute disgrace I am. I have failed again.*

I have lost count of how many times this scenario has played out in my life. Way too many. And it really is like torture. Great hope built up for a great new future and then great despair over dreams crushed yet again.

And the honest truth is that this is still a work in progress for me. It's still a day-to-day thing. I am still figuring it out. My main goal has become to be aware of patterns and try to figure out what the triggers are and to be a witness to them instead of mindlessly going through the motions of my life. Why do I believe this new diet will work? Why do I want to eat this entire cake? Why was I able to breeze through today without a single craving? Why do I feel the urge to stuff my face? Why do I feel good? Why do I feel bad? And so on and so on.

Along the line somewhere I started noticing trends with my eating habits and my overall well-being. I started realizing that my current mental status and emotional health were in direct correlation to my current body shape and size. I realized that my outward appearance was a direct reflection of my inner well-being. I have noticed that so many factors play into what I am eating and how I am feeling. Aha!

I started making a list. When do I feel like binging? What is going on in my life when I feel good and don't even feel hungry? What is going on in my life when I feel like I am starving and I want to eat a dozen donuts? What does my life look like when I am trim and healthy? What does my life look like when I am obese and at my lowest?

I have, by no means, won this battle quite yet. But I have lost weight and I have made significant progress in my obsessive battle with food. That's what I will be sharing with you. I wrote this book to share with you what I have come to realize about the correlation between my body size and the rest of my life. This book is not only about food. It's about building a life in which you don't even want to binge. It's about building a life that is free from the obsession of food. It's about nurturing your inner world which will, in most cases, have a positive effect on your outward appearance.

The chapters in this book are ordered in a way that seemed to make sense to me. I want you to start at the beginning and work your way through without skipping anything or jumping around. I promise you that it will pay off.

Oh, and here's a surprise. The chapter on what to eat is the very last chapter. Why? Because I believe that the chapters that come before are where the real weight loss magic happens.

I really wish you the best on your journey. This food battle is no joke and I absolutely understand how hard it is. I hope this book helps you find some peace with it.

Chapter 1: *The Story*

Here's a little story for you. Enjoy.

Day 1:

<u>7:15am</u>: Today is the day! I am starting my new life today! I feel motivated, excited, and so

hopeful. Oh, yeah!! I am PUMPED! I am absolutely positive that, THIS TIME, the diet will work. Why? Because I have (yet again) reached the point where I cannot take one more single second of being fat. I have reached the point where the pain of being overweight exceeds the pleasure of eating whatever I want.

And, let's be honest, I feel disgusted with myself. My body aches, my clothes are too tight, and I feel ashamed. I am too embarrassed to even go to lunch with friends because I am so fat. I want to stay home and hide.

That being said, there is no other option than to stick to this diet and lose the damn weight. So I am excited! I just know I can do it this time. I want it SO bad. I want, more than anything, to be thin. I want to feel good in my clothes. I want to live my life without having it revolve around food. I want to be able to go anywhere I want and do anything I want without having to feel anxiety about how I look. I want to be invited to a party and not have my first thought be, *oh dear God I cannot go to this party because I haven't lost the weight and I look like a whale in all my clothes.*

How nice it would be to get invited to a party and, instead, think to myself, *hmmmm, that sounds like a fun party, maybe I'll go.* I can't even fathom that. I can't wrap my head around making life choices that don't take into consideration my current weight. And that, my friends, makes me horribly sad.

So here I sit ready to head full speed into another diet. And the honest truth is that I feel sick to my stomach and I have a headache. I feel hungover. Why? Because, in celebration of starting my new life today, I spent all of yesterday afternoon and evening stuffing my face. Literally. I ate anything and everything in sight because I knew that today things are changing. Marshmallows, cake pops, cheeseburger and fries, chocolate, cookies, Rice Krispie treats. All of it. Every last bite. Until I was nauseated.

Day 2:

8:58am: Okay, day one was a success! I stuck to eating well. It was pretty easy. Well, it was bound to be pretty easy because it was day one and my motivation was through the roof. I am still feeling highly motivated today so I assume today will go pretty easily as well. I already feel a little smaller. Even just one day of cutting way back on sugary carbs can make me feel smaller. I mean, I was up all night peeing but whatever. I would rather be up all night peeing than spend one more day feeling ginormous.

<u>4:24pm</u>: Well, I am not going to lie. Here we are on the afternoon of day number two and I am already wanting to cheat. I am tired and nothing sounds better or more comforting right now than a pizza and then some dessert. God, it would just taste and feel so good. But I am going to try to say no. I am going to try my hardest to breathe my way through this and resist.

Day 3:

<u>10:23am</u>: Okay, I cheated. I did great all day yesterday and then, by about 6 PM, I just couldn't resist having a cookie. I did good and only ate one. And then I had a good, healthy dinner. And then everything went downhill. Ugh. I had about six big sugar cookies. Sheesh. I mean, they tasted REALLY good. But I am back on track this morning and I just know it's going to be a good day.

Day 4:

<u>7:36am</u>: I feel sick. I feel depressed and angry with myself. I did okay yesterday and then completely lost it last night. I ate a bunch of bread. I ate marshmallows and chocolate. And today I feel sad. I feel sick to my stomach, bloated, and defeated. I want to kick myself. WHAT IS WRONG WITH ME??? I see so

many people who are so capable of being so disciplined and I just literally can't even last a few days. It's like food is a drug to me. I can't resist the urge. I lose all control for a few minutes of bliss and then I feel horrible, even worse, than I did before. I can't go on like this. I feel miserable. I feel worthless.

Day 5:

<u>6:05am</u>: I give up.

Sound familiar?

I don't know what your story involves but mine goes something like this. Diet. Binge. Diet. Binge. Diet. Binge. Hate myself. Be excited about a new diet. Hate myself. Repeat. For thirty or so years.

For as long as I can remember, I have been obsessed with my weight. Either losing it, gaining it, or somewhere in between. But never really satisfied. Always wishing and hoping and struggling.

To be honest, for most of my life, I couldn't even imagine a life that didn't involve obsessing over my weight. I couldn't even fathom the idea of living my life free from constant thoughts of whether or not I look fat. Oh, you mean to tell me there are people on this Earth who don't spend all their waking hours trying to figure out how to get thinner? Obviously, they are aliens, or they have some sort of missing gene. I mean, that's just WEIRD.

Anyway, the majority of my adult life has involved some sort of diet or weight loss regimen. I have been fat, skinny, large, small, pudgy, obese, thin, and everything in between. No days off for this girl. Weight loss and dieting have been the one constant for the better part of my almost fifty years. Yikes.

Several years ago, I found myself a divorced, overweight, forty-something mom. I found myself in the depths of one of my life's darkest times. I was nothing short of miserable. I was fat, broke, exhausted, lonely, angry, and down in the dumps. I needed a complete life overhaul. I needed to make some drastic changes.

Of course, one of these changes involved losing weight. So, as per my usual tactics, I set out to try the latest diet. I tried keto. I tried paleo. I tried intermittent fasting. I tried juice fasting. I tried the diets with the little packets of "food." I tried ALL OF THEM. And, don't get me wrong, for a bit of time they worked. I would initially drop some weight and feel really great. But, inevitably, starvation, or a stressful event at work, or a series of exhausting days would set in and I would, once again, bail on the diet. I would abandon the diet, soothe my starving tummy with cookies, pizza, and ice cream, and then hate myself. Over and over again. Same story, different day. For years!

Somewhere along the way, I started working on my self-esteem. I started really diving into making changes. I started thinking differently and trying out new ways of living and eating. I started looking at food differently.

And, you know what? I started breaking free. I started losing my obsession with dieting. I started actually losing weight! I know, literally sounds impossible, right? It's not. I promise you.

This book is my attempt to do my best to pass on to you everything I have learned in my almost fifty years of weight struggles. I am going to do my best to help you break free from the trap of weight loss obsession. I am going to do my best to help you actually, once and for all, lose the damn weight.

First, we will consider some possible reasons you may be carrying extra weight. And then I am going to walk you through the specific steps I used to lose the weight and break free from the diet/binge cycle of Hell.

Are you ready? Let's go.

Chapter 2: *What is Your Body Trying to Tell You?*

Eight years ago I got divorced. The years immediately following my divorce were a roller coaster ride of emotions, good times and horrible times, extreme sadness, unexpected bliss, crushing loneliness, freedom, massive debt, relentless fear, hope, and inevitable transformation. It was no less than chaos. All of this while trying to be the best mom I could be to my two amazing kids. I was literally living my life one day at a time and, most days, couldn't even tell you what day of the week it was. Ugh. Needless to say, I had other things to think about besides my body and my health. And, sure enough, all it took was one look at my physical appearance to give you a glimpse into my internal world.

Prior to my divorce, I was fit, trim, and athletic. I ate somewhat healthily, exercised most days, and I even participated regularly in marathons and triathlons. And all of this showed in my outward appearance. I was thin and sun-kissed and healthy looking.

Well, cut to my post-divorce years and my outward appearance was drastically different. I quit exercising (I didn't have time to), I gained thirty pounds, I had bags under my eyes, and I was pale from lack of sunshine. Ugh. And, needless to say, I was depressed, grumpy, and angry. Yikes. I felt AWFUL.

I started becoming so ashamed of myself and I quit wanting to leave my house. I basically became a hermit. My whole life revolved around my kids and work. Nothing else. No exercise. No girls' nights out. No days at the spa. No good nights of sleep. Nothing. Instead, I was doing long carpool lines, stressful shifts at work, fast-food meals, late nights, early mornings, Netflix marathons, and mouthfuls of soothing, numbing cookies and cupcakes. Oof. You get the picture. I quickly packed on a whopping THIRTY pounds. I quickly went from trim and sun-kissed to strung out, tired, and frumpy. I hated myself. I was so ashamed of myself.

What is the point of me telling you this? Well, it seems to me that the assumption can easily be made that our outward appearance and our inward state of affairs can be directly correlated. Okay, I get it, you may be thinking to yourself, *That's so obvious!!!* But hear me out. I think it goes a lot deeper than just the idea that being stressed out, depressed, and tired leads to being overweight, frumpy, and haggard looking. Let's look a little deeper.

What if we started looking at the actual mental processes that may be going on in your life? Are you post-divorce? Okay, would it not be a stretch to say you may be carrying some baggage? And I don't just mean emotional baggage. Could you possibly be carrying some anger that's conveniently disguised as extra fat on your thighs? Could you possibly be carrying some unresolved grief disguised as those pesky love handles? I believe so. So maybe those extra stomach rolls are more symbolic than just a matter of eating too many bon-bons on Saturday night.

Let's go even deeper. Immediately after I divorced, I jumped right on into the dating pool. Ugh. This was not my best idea. I was still an emotional mess. I was still dealing with ex issues. I was still trying to find my way through grief and pain. But, nevertheless, I jumped in anyway.

Well, after a year or two of heartache, stress, and dating disasters, I decided that I needed a little break. Well, let me be honest, I didn't really consciously decide to take a break from dating. The universe decided for me. Men no longer showed up and asked me out. Nobody that I knew made any more requests to set me up on dates with people they knew. Essentially, it was like I was officially taken out of the dating pool. And, to be honest, this was fine by me. I was convinced that dating and relationships only led to heartbreak. I felt like I was doomed to be alone for the rest of my life.

This was around the time that I started my hermit phase and started packing on the pounds. I started focusing all my attention on my kids and my job. I spent my weekends either hanging with the kids or, when they were at their dad's house,

I would stay home and watch Netflix, or clean my house, or drive to the shopping center in the next town over so that I didn't have to see anyone I knew. I didn't want anyone seeing me in the shape I was in. I was so ashamed. My only comfort and joy came from my children and donuts. Ouch.

This phase of my life went on for a few years. During this time, I would periodically long for a companion and I would wish I had a boyfriend to spend time together with. I longed for love and I daydreamed of the day a great guy would walk into my life.

Here's the kicker. I would constantly say to myself, *If I just lose this weight and get myself together, then I will be ready to put myself back out there.* The weight I was carrying was the ONE reason I didn't put myself back out there and give dating a try once again. It was the only thing holding me back from being more social and saying yes to party invitations, lunch invites, and any other potential activities that may have led to me meeting someone. I repeatedly used the excuse of my weight to keep on being a hermit.

And what's bananas is that, over the course of time that I was overweight and miserable and wishing I had a boyfriend, I was constantly dieting and putting myself through awful cycles of starving and binging. I was trying every diet known to man. But nothing "worked". Sure, I would lose some weight initially. But then, inevitably, I would abandon the diet and that weight would creep back on. Oftentimes bringing more weight along with it. It was a never-ending cycle of starve, lose, binge, gain. Ugh. It was MISERABLE.

But what's interesting is that I kept thinking to myself that I still couldn't put myself into the dating world until I did lose the darn weight. Even though I repeatedly tried and was unsuccessful. Even though I seemingly wanted a relationship so badly. I was convinced that I was trying so hard to lose this weight so that I could start dating again, but that I was just unable to lose it. Like, as if there were some cosmic forces that were blocking me from losing it. As if I was giving it 100% but there was just something wrong with me and I was destined to be fat and lonely the rest of my life. I was absolutely positive that I was doing everything in my power to lose weight and that I was just unlucky or had some sort of fat gene that was preventing me from being successful. Ugh.

Like I said before, this went on for a few years. Meanwhile, my kids were growing up. My son graduated from high school and then my daughter. During this time, I started really thinking about the idea of dating again. The idea of my kids leaving home and the subsequent quiet house that that would bring made me really aware of my singleness. I was dreading my kids leaving home as it was and to think of them leaving combined with me being single had me envisioning myself on a deserted island writing "SEND HELP" in the sand. Yikes.

So, as we spent the summer before my daughter left for college packing and preparing, I came to the decision that, as scary and dreadful as it sounded, I wanted to open myself back up to the idea of dating. I wanted to be in a relationship again. I asked myself the same questions I previously had and, this time, I was able to say that I was still scared but now willing to take my chances and start thinking about putting myself back out there. I was able to truthfully answer "yes" to the questions of dating, sharing my life, and risking my heart. This time I answered with a shaky, but solid, "YES" and not a "yeah, sure, sounds good".

I know, this probably sounds like a coping mechanism for me dealing with my daughter leaving. And, honestly, knowing me, it most certainly was. But, whatever. It's how I felt at the time. Anyway, the point is, once I consciously decided that I definitely wanted to try dating again, the weight actually started coming off. The healthy eating actually "worked". I set my mind to eating a clean, healthy, doable way of eating and I started seeing the numbers on the scale drop. No starvation. No crazy fad dieting. No expensive meal plans. Just honest to goodness clean, healthy eating. The scale started moving down! I actually started to lose weight! Finally!

So, what was going on here? Why did the weight start coming off now? Why did I find it easier to stick to my healthy plan? What had changed? At first glance, it appeared that nothing had changed. But then I started really thinking about it.

Looking back over the last few years, what had changed in regards to my thoughts about dating? As in, thinking about what dating would be like and thinking about what it would be like to have a man in my life. How would that feel? How would my daily life change? How would my priorities change? And so on.

This is when I came to a scary realization. Asking these questions of myself really got me thinking. Over the past few years, or really since I got divorced, had I really ever wanted to be in a relationship? Had I really and truly wanted to date again? Had I really wanted to risk heartache all over? Had I really wanted to give my time to anyone other than my kids? Had I really been willing to share my Christmases with anyone other than my kids?

Much to my surprise, I found myself answering these questions with a big fat "NO". What??? How had I thought for YEARS that I wanted to date again and thought for YEARS that the one and only reason I was not in a relationship was my weight? How had I been convinced that the only reason I was unattached was because I was fat? How had I been so sure that the weight was the only thing keeping me from what I was so sure that I wanted?

Coming to this realization that maybe I had subconsciously been avoiding relationships this whole time and consciously blaming it on my weight was the eye opener I really needed. I realized that I had never truly asked myself what I really, actually wanted and, honestly, maybe I really didn't even consciously know what I wanted.

For all those years, I THOUGHT I wanted to be in a relationship. I thought that I was just being held back by my weight. I thought that I would be okay sharing my life with someone besides my kids. But, in reality, I had never truly asked myself those questions and never truly acknowledged the true answers to them. The true answer would have been that, even though I felt lonely and longed for companionship, I was not willing to share my life with anyone besides my kids. Even though I thought that it would have been so nice to have someone to go to movies with and talk about my day with, I was not yet ready to risk my heart again. Even though I really missed having a partner, I was not yet willing to face dating again. Oof. That's a big realization to come to. But it's also a gateway to freedom.

I realized that there was a real possibility that maybe I was subconsciously sabotaging my dieting to stay single. What? Yep. I realized that my weight that I fought against so strongly, was actually PROTECTING me from what I, deep down, knew I did not actually want. I fully came to understand that my weight was my subconscious protector. My weight was my excuse. My weight was my defense. My weight was cushioning me from any potential pain. My weight was protecting me from having to risk my heart again. My weight was my armor.

After lots of thought, I came to the realization that I may have, all along, been actually keeping myself plump in an effort to stay where I was. I may have been sabotaging the very body that I knew might lead to me going on dates. I was, most definitely, sabotaging my weight loss efforts to remain single and avoid having to do anything that involved being away from my kids. The truth is that staying single was scary also. But it was far less scary than dating.

What might your weight be protecting you from? After I came to this realization and gave it some serious thought, I concluded that our weight can be our means of defense against anything. Good or bad.

Maybe you really want to take that vacation but, deep down, it feels scary so you keep telling yourself that you are too fat for the airplane seat. Maybe you really want that new job in marketing but a big career move feels really overwhelming so, instead, you keep on telling yourself that you are too fat to wear the cute, trendy outfits that would be required. Maybe you, like I did, believe you really want to find your Prince Charming, but you're terrified of another rejection so you tell yourself that the only reason you haven't is because you can't yet fit into those skinny jeans. Might you be avoiding making the scary decision to leave a bad relationship, but you tell yourself that you are staying because you could never find another partner since you are fat?

What could possibly be some other reasons behind your avoidance of these things? If you took away your excuse of being overweight, what reasons would you find for not going ahead and doing these things? Maybe you are actually scared of change. Maybe you actually aren't mentally ready for a new relationship. Maybe moving away feels horrifying. Maybe you like spending all your time with your kids and don't want to give that up. Maybe you feel like you couldn't possibly endure one more rejection.

Finding the answers to these questions may require some serious introspection and real honesty. It's super easy to use weight as an excuse and avoid looking deeper.

Also, to be completely honest, if you are significantly overweight, using weight as an excuse really is the perfect avoidance tactic because it buys you time. You can't just take off fifty pounds overnight. I mean, I guess you could have a leg surgically removed but that's not what we are talking about here! So, even if you dive deep and acknowledge what your true feelings and reasons may be, you still have to do the work and take the time to lose the weight. So you still have a "cushion" of time to face your fears about what it is you want to do. If it takes six months to lose fifty pounds, then that is six months of time that you can spend mentally preparing and readying yourself for whatever it is that you want to accomplish. Seems to me that this makes carrying an extra fifty pounds the perfect way to avoid things because it buys you at least six months of time.

So, what might you be buying time for? What might you be avoiding? What might you be protecting yourself from? What decision might you fear making so, instead, you are creating an excuse for?

Let's look at another scenario. Let's take a minute and think about boundaries. Are you good at saying no when you mean no? Are you good at speaking up for yourself? Are you good at voicing your feelings and opinions? Yes? No? Well, if you are anything like me, this is an area that requires constant improvement. Oof.

I used to be, to put it bluntly, a welcome mat. Come on in! Step right on me! Wipe your feet! I can take it! I had no sense of boundaries and I was like a people pleaser on steroids. Your wish was my command. If you needed anything at all, I was your girl. You needed a glass of water while

I was fighting for my life in the ICU? No problem! Let me just check myself out of the hospital and run right over! You need to whine about your wrinkled duvet cover while I am going through divorce, bankruptcy, foreclosure, and my car just died? Sure! Let me drop everything and lend you an ear! You are mad because I said no to a dinner date when I am exhausted from working eleven days in a row and have a child at home with fever? I get it! I should feel horribly guilty for turning down your invitation! Yikes.

Needless to say, I used to have a real problem with setting boundaries and sticking up for myself. So, you know what I did instead? I stuffed all of those ignored feelings down. Every single time that I said yes when I really meant no, I would subsequently stuff down the "no" that was screaming to be let out of me. I would stuff it down with donuts. I would stifle it with pizza. I would quiet it with cookies. My wants, needs, feelings, and boundaries were all screaming to be released but I could not let them out. I feared confrontation. I feared rejection. I feared not being loved. So instead, I stuffed it all down. I carried every single "no" in my hips. I lugged around all my denied needs in my stomach rolls. I toted around all my wishy-washy boundaries in my squishy bottom. I comforted my internal cries for acknowledgment with warm cookies and mouth-watering chips and queso.

This also extended to expressing my emotions in all my relationships. Coworker relationships. Family relationships. Romantic relationships. The girl at the grocery cash register relationships. All of them.

I used to put on a sunny face for all these people and pretend like nothing was ever wrong and every day was the best day ever. I was like Mary Poppins. Me, angry? Never! Me, sad? No way! Me, disappointed? Absolutely not! I did my best to completely deny that I ever experienced negative emotions. I did my best to completely ignore any trace of bad feelings.

Well, you can imagine how successful this was. Turns out, much to my surprise, that ignored feelings and emotions don't just disappear off the face of the Earth. Shocker! Those pesky little things like to be acknowledged and felt. And, even more surprisingly, turns out that, if you just go ahead and acknowledge and feel them, they go away! I know, crazy, right? Well, this was a lesson that I took my sweet, old time learning. Ugh.

For as long as I can remember, I was a confrontation avoider. I had the hardest time speaking up for myself and I rarely was able to work up the courage to speak my mind and express my feelings. Instead, I usually acted embarrassingly passive-aggressive. Eww. Or I completely distanced myself from people instead of having a conversation. Eww again. I just couldn't figure out how to speak up. It felt impossible to me and like I had somehow missed out on the gene required for expressing feelings. Ugh.

So, you guessed it, instead of conveying my feelings like a mature adult, I ate them. And, you guessed it again, I wore them in the form of cellulite. Oh, is that anger I see on your hips? Sure is! Pardon me, but is that frustration and fear I see bulging out from your skinny jeans? Yep! Oh my, you sure have a lot of sadness pouring over the top of your bra strap. I sure do! Yikes. You get the picture. My point here is that stuffing ANYTHING down, whether it be emotions or pizza, is going to make the numbers on the scale go up. The only way out of this tornado is to stop stuffing.

And don't go thinking that these emotions we may be carrying around in our bulging waistlines have to be current emotions. They indeed do not. That extra roll around your stomach? Could be that stuffed down shame from that time in 1982 when your pants ripped in front of the entire class. That double chin you hate so much? Could be that pent up anger from that time when your college roommate slept with your boyfriend. Yikes. And those love handles that you despise? Could be remnants of the abandonment you felt when your parents divorced and your mom left. Sigh. My point is, we carry all this junk around with us until we deal with it. I once heard it described this way by the author, Mastin Kipp, and this is when it all clicked for me. He said, "the issues are in the tissues". Holy guacamole. That's some serious truth.

What would change about your perspective if you knew that your extra weight is directly related to your emotional "baggage"? Would you, perhaps, change the way you try to lose weight? Maybe come at it from a different angle? Would you possibly even shift your focus from the food you consume to working on healing your inner self? Hmmm.

A few years ago, I decided it was time to put my life back together after my divorce and start rebuilding my self-esteem. I read multiple self-help books. I went to therapy. I did all the things.

Gradually, my self-esteem started improving. I started actually believing that I might kind of be a somewhat worthy person. I quit beating myself up for literally everything and I started being a little more compassionate with myself.

Well, low and behold, guess what happened? I started catching myself speaking up for myself! It was like a freaking miracle! I started catching myself taking baby steps towards saying no when I meant no. Hallelujah! I started to let that irritating coworker know when she had crossed the line. I started ignoring people expecting me to be a doormat. I started speaking up when someone had crossed one of my boundaries. I quit answering the phone calls of those friends who wanted to take advantage of my doormat nature. And, here's the greatest part, I found myself binging on cookies far less often! I found myself being able to feel the anger, express it, and be done with it. No stuffing required. Amazing!

Now, don't get me wrong. This is definitely a baby steps process and I still struggle with this on the daily. But I have definitely made progress and this has definitely made a world of difference in my tendency to overeat cake. It really has.

My conclusion has been that the stronger the emotion that doesn't get released, the bigger the binge there is likely to be. My conclusion is that:

Extreme anxiety = extreme ice cream sundaes.
Extreme anger = extreme amounts of cookies.
Extreme inability to speak up = extreme pizza

And so on.

Another interesting thing to point out is that I have found that, personally, anxiety and anger seem to be the most triggering emotions in relation to potential binges. For some reason, comfort foods really are comforting when it comes to anxiety (stress) and anger. That being said, it might be helpful to pay close attention to times when you are experiencing these emotions and actively take measures to work through them instead of stuffing them down.

So, in summary, what might your weight be telling you? What might your weight represent? What might your weight be protecting you from? What might your weight be helping you to avoid?

It may be helpful to sit down, or take a walk, or take a drive in your car and think about these things. As they say, knowledge is power. If you find that some of the above scenarios are relevant to you, then you can start figuring out what to do about it.

Are you avoiding doing something? Well, how can you work to acknowledge that your weight may actually just be your armor? Can you start speaking your truth and free yourself to take off the armor? Do you have trouble expressing anger? Maybe you can start working on your self-esteem so that you feel more comfortable expressing your feelings. Do you suffer from anxiety that you quell with comfort foods? Maybe you can start incorporating more stress relieving measures into your life to reduce your anxiety levels.

Next, I want to touch on another aspect of our mental states. Something interesting that I have found is that the words and feelings we use to describe our lives are oftentimes surprisingly telling when it comes to the state of our body. Let's explore this.

Here's a quick exercise for you. Get out a pen and piece of paper. Stop everything you are doing right now and focus on thinking about your life. I want you to focus on the adjectives that you would use to describe your current life. Not just your body but your life and everything in it. Your relationships. Your job. Your home. Your family. Your hobbies. Your spirituality. Your friends. All of it.

Okay, now I want you to, quickly and without much thought or judgment, write down every single word that comes to mind when you think of your current life. Write them all down.

Got them down? Okay, now we are going to go word by word and try to imagine how each word might correlate to our current physical body. I am going to show you how the words you use to describe your life can be very telling.

Here's an example for you. Your paper may look something like this:

Unfulfilled = hungry, empty (need to be filled)
Happy = filled, light, vibrant
Bored = need entertainment (food/other vices)
Stuck = unable to change current status (weight)
Depressed = heavy (literally)
Stressed = weighed down (literally)
Scared = need protection/armor (weight)
Anxious = need comfort (comfort foods)
Exhausted/depleted = need to be filled (food)
Fulfilled = don't need to be filled, satisfied
Angry = need soothing (comfort foods)
Lonely = empty/need more (food)
Filled with love = nurtured (healthy food)
Hate = punishment (starve/binge/purge/etc.)
Guilt = punishment (starve/binge/purge/etc.)
Joyful = filled, full, not in need (of food)

Do you see how this works? These are just a few of the many examples of words we could use to describe our current mental states and how they may be related to our current physical states. The most important conclusion that I can draw from this is that working on improving ALL aspects of our life is a super important piece of the weight loss puzzle. I would argue that any attempts you make to lose weight are pretty much doomed if you are living in a state of anger, stress, or guilt.

What it all comes down to is that your extra weight is usually not just about the sleeve of cookies you ate on Tuesday night. Your extra pounds are not just a matter of you being "lazy" or lacking willpower. Those extra pounds are, quite often, a metaphor for what's really going on inside of you. That bulge on your waistline might just be a glimpse into your true feelings. That higher number on the scale might really be a sign of your current need for armor.

What is your body trying to tell you?

Chapter 3: *What Are You Telling Your Body?*

We just took a close look at clues your body may be trying to give you. Now let's switch gears and look at what you may be telling your body. What on Earth do I mean? Hang on and you'll see. Let's take a look.

Several years ago, I heard a story about a girl who had been in one physically abusive relationship after the other. I, of course, felt horrified for her but it also made me wonder why any woman would continue to suffer through such traumatic relationships. Why didn't she leave? I wondered what was going on inside of her to make her believe that she deserved to be treated in this horrendous way.

This is when someone explained to me the concept of "guilt seeks punishment." From my understanding, on some sort of subconscious level, if you feel guilty for something, you will subconsciously seek out situations in which you are punished. Essentially, the idea is that, on some sort of subconscious level, this woman may have believed, for whatever reason, that she deserved to be "punished."

How sad and horrifying is that? I don't know if this is true or not, but this was how it was explained to me. And I am not sure I am a fan of this idea because it almost makes it sound like it's HER fault that she is being abused. No way. But, anyway, we can definitely all agree that this is nightmarish.

To further expand, another component of this type of situation is that the "guilt" the woman may be subconsciously feeling that is, in turn, subconsciously seeking "punishment" was, most likely, given to her by her abuser. What does this mean? Well, it means that, through disgusting tactics such as gaslighting and emotional/verbal abuse, the abuser has convinced the woman (or man!!!) that they are somehow the one to blame. The abuser has projected all his (or her!!!) guilt onto the abused. So the abused party is, most likely, subconsciously taking on guilt that doesn't even belong to them! Now, if that doesn't fire you up, then I don't know what will! It's the classic story of an abuser telling his or her victim that they "made" them do it because of their bad behavior. Very sad.

So, what on Earth does this have to do with weight loss?? Well, what if we take a quick look at some of the possible beliefs you hold about yourself and how they may be influencing how you treat your body and how this affects your eating.

Let's consider the "guilt seeks punishment" theory. What could this possibly look like in relation to dieting?

Well, what if I make up a possible scenario for this. Let's say you are fifty pounds overweight. And let's say your unhealthy eating has spiraled out of control. Maybe you have been really stressed about work and you are short on time. Or maybe you have a new baby and you are literally exhausted and can't hold your eyes open.

Or maybe you are in the process of moving and you have been consumed with packing, cleaning, arranging, and planning. No matter the issue, the point is that you have a lot going on and your eating habits have fallen to the bottom of your priority list. Maybe you have been getting by on fast food and pizza deliveries for the past month.

Well, one day, in the midst of the chaos, you stop and take a good, long look in the mirror. What do you see? Chances are you see a version of yourself that you are not happy with. Chances are you see a fluffier version of yourself and quite possibly a more frazzled, unkempt version of yourself. How does this make you feel? Well, I would guess that this makes you feel pretty crappy. I would also guess that this instantly makes you regret the last month's worth of Chinese takeout and convenience store donuts. What happens next?

My bet would be that there's a pretty good chance that you are going to start beating yourself up. I know that's how I would typically have handled this situation. I would instantly feel regret and then start berating myself for being such a horrible person. I would bash myself for being lazy, gluttonous, and lacking willpower. And then what? I would immediately start planning my next starvation diet. I would immediately tell myself that tomorrow I would start the beginning of a five-day juice fast, or a ten-day carrots-only diet, or any other strict, low calorie, torture diet. Ugh.

Do you see what's happening here? I engaged in behavior that I judged as "wrong," so I considered myself "guilty" and, subsequently, deserving of "punishment." Interesting, huh?

Would it be a stretch to say that the whole never-ending diet/binge cycle could be linked to a "bad" behavior = "guilt" = "punishment" cycle? Hmmm. Just a thought.

Think about it this way. You binge on junk food ("bad" behavior). You then feel guilty and mentally beat yourself up. You then tell your body that it deserves to be punished through starvation. Sounds pretty harsh, doesn't it?

I want to stop here and point out that this is where the absolute, undeniable importance of self-love and self-compassion come in. When you get to the level of truly having these two things, you no longer find yourself capable of "punishing" yourself. You no longer believe you are "guilty" or deserving of being treated badly. You start to believe that you are a human being deserving of grace and understanding and love.

You start to believe that you deserve to be treated well. At this point, all these punishing type behaviors cease to exist. You no longer feel the need to beat yourself up for anything. Pretty amazing, huh? More on this later!

Okay, so back to the topic of what we may be telling our bodies. Let's dive even deeper into the example above.

When you decide that you have been "bad" and you need to starve yourself, what else might you be telling your body? Well, maybe you are telling your body that it doesn't deserve nourishment. Or maybe that it doesn't deserve to be taken care of. Most likely you are conveying to your body that it deserves to be starved, tortured, and beaten up. Sounds crazy, right? But seriously think about it. When you put your body through such harsh diet regimens, this is exactly the message you are conveying. Ouch. Makes me want to give myself a big hug.

What if we took this idea and expanded it beyond the scope of just our eating habits? What if we applied this to other areas of our life or our current mental state of affairs? Are there areas of your life in which you feel guilty? Is there something else going on in your life for which you believe you deserve to be punished for? If the answer is yes, what can you do to start processing these issues and working on forgiving yourself? How can you resolve these issues so that they no longer show up in your life in sneaky little ways like the food you are putting on your plate?

I have found that, quite often, everyone has past events that we feel some sort of guilt about. These things just sit in the backs of our minds, festering and causing problems until we face them.

We can feel guilty for small things, like the time in fifth grade when we accidentally stepped on Jenny's foot and made her cry. Or we can feel guilty for much bigger things, like putting our kids through a divorce. Either way, these things stay with us until we deal with them. Instead of letting them fester on and ride around on our hips like baggage, we really need to address them and be done with them. A lot of the times, if you can address the memories of the guilt you have and give the situation a second look, you can reframe it into a different story that doesn't create a feeling of guilt that you have to carry around.

Let me give you a quick example of this ridiculous thing I used to feel guilty about. When I was a teenager, I went on a vacation with my dad. We were out sightseeing and riding on one of those hop on/hop off buses. We loaded onto the bus and, as the tour guide announced we were about to depart and was giving a quick talk about our next stop, my dad jumped off the bus to snap one last photo. Well, as he was taking the picture, the bus started to slowly pull away. I panicked. I knew my dad was off the bus. I was in the very back of the bus and I was scared and mortified and didn't know what to do. Suddenly, the lady sitting next to me yelled, "your dad! He's not on the bus!" The bus stopped and my dad, who had run alongside, hopped back on with no problems. The event was over. But, you know what? For YEARS, I felt guilty about this. I felt guilty because I had not been the one to speak up. I felt guilty because I panicked and I was embarrassed. I felt guilty because it made me wonder what would have happened if that lady didn't speak up. Would I have ever spoken up? Would I have just left my dad behind? What kind of human does that? Ugh. Anyway, for years this memory sat in the back of my mind and every time I thought of it, I cringed with guilt.

And then something happened. One day I thought of it again. This time I really thought about it. It occurred to me that just maybe I wasn't the only "guilty" person here. Looking back, my dad shouldn't have jumped off the bus!

After all, we had all loaded back on and the driver had already announced that we were leaving. So, he really shouldn't have gotten off! I was left in a position to have to stop the bus just for him. And that's not necessarily a fair position to be put in. So, my point is, as it turns out, I wasn't the only guilty party in this scenario. And for goodness' sake, I was a teenager! Of course I was mortified by my dad's goofy behavior! That's how teenagers are! Considering my age, I was just being NORMAL.

So, what's the lesson here? The memories that we carry around with us and feel guilty about can, oftentimes, be revisited and reframed into new memories that don't cause such negative feelings and remorse.

What memories that you maybe feel guilty for, or bad about, can you rethink and try to reframe? What old memories can you reconsider and give yourself some grace for? Oftentimes, our memories are still seen from the vantage point of a child or younger person. Therefore, the memories are, most likely, being viewed from the mind of an immature and/or not-yet-wise child or young adult. Why does this matter? Well, when you go back and look at the situation from a grownup's perspective, you can see that your fears, concerns, and feelings may have been unjustified. This can be extremely freeing. When you truly free yourself from the chains of guilt, it just may show up in the form of what you put on your plate.

Fine, you might be saying, *but what about things I have done as an adult? What about that time three years ago when I screamed at my kid for spilling the milk?* Well, firstly, who hasn't screamed at their kids at least a gagillion times? We ALL do things like this and then feel HORRIBLE afterwards. So, how can you reframe this awful memory? Well, what if you just gave yourself some grace about it? What if you remind yourself that you may have been exhausted or depressed or all of the above? What if you reminded yourself that parents are just humans trying to do the best they can? And, most importantly, we all make mistakes and that doesn't make us bad, guilty people. It just means we had a rough moment. No more, no less. And the fact that you even carry guilt about this means that you are, indeed, an awesome parent! And I would bet my tiny bank account that your kids still think you hung the moon. For real.

Let's look at another way we tell our bodies stories. Have you ever considered the idea of quitting dieting completely and then thought to yourself, *oh no, there is NO WAY I could be trusted to just eat whatever I want!*. I know I used to think this all of the time. I truly believed that I had no control over my eating and I would, most likely, eat myself to death if left unattended at a buffet. Yikes. I believed that I couldn't trust myself and needed to be controlled when it came to eating. So how did this show up in my life? Strict, controlled diets that allowed for no mistakes. I needed to have complete control over every bite that went into my mouth or else the floodgates might open and I would cycle into an out of control binge. Oof. I didn't trust myself in the slightest. Sound familiar?

On the flip side, let's consider binging. Because, as we all know, every diet is followed by a binge. Well, if you inherently believe that you are not trustworthy, wouldn't it make sense that you would end every diet with a binge? I mean, it's the ultimate validation, right? It's like you are saying, "See, I was right all along! I can't be trusted! I always fail!" Ugh. How sad is that? And then, what do you do? Yep, you guessed it. You punish yourself for being untrustworthy. You start a new strict diet. And the cycle goes on and on forever.

What if we apply this idea to other aspects of our life? In other areas of your life, do you trust yourself? Do you trust yourself in relationships?

Do you trust yourself at work? More specifically, do you trust YOU to take care of YOU?

This is an area in which I have often found myself lacking. It has occurred to me that I didn't trust myself at all to take care of myself. Why? I had a track record of abandoning my own needs in an effort to please others. I had a track record of deserting my own needs. I had a track record of not being trustworthy when it came to me. What did this look like? Maybe I would say yes when I really meant no. Maybe I would say I was fine when I really wasn't. Maybe I would abandon my plans to go to the gym when work asked me to stay late. Maybe I would give up on my goal when things got tough. All these examples led me to feel that I couldn't trust me. I believed that I was untrustworthy and could only be counted on to abandon myself. And, you guessed it, this showed up in the way I ate. I couldn't trust myself with food. I needed to be controlled.

Let me give you a current times example of what not trusting yourself and/or abandoning yourself might look like. Currently there's a pandemic going on. Not news to you, I'm sure. Good old COVID-19. Well, as many of you know, this virus has turned out to be a great divider. People all over the world have formed their opinions on all aspects of this virus and how it should be handled. People have opinions on masks. People have opinions on vaccines. People have opinions on EVERYTHING. Phew. Well, why am I bringing this up? Because this may be a good time to look at some examples of how you could potentially be abandoning yourself.

Let's say, for example, that you have read the data and you believe that masks are necessary to stop the spread of the virus. You believe that the masks are effective and, therefore, you avoid taking them off in public because you fear that you might be exposed to the virus. This is your belief and it is based on your research, your feelings, and your concerns. This is your personal decision. You don't care whether other people wear one, but for you, a mask it is. You believe you are doing the right thing by wearing the mask. Okay, got it?

Well, now let's say you run into your old high school crush at the gas station. He is still SO dreamy. You stop to say hello and catch up. He does not have a mask on. Shortly into the conversation he says something like, "you are wearing one of those stupid masks?? Those are useless!! You really should take that ridiculous thing off!!".

You immediately feel super awkward, a little embarrassed, and, quite frankly, bullied. You literally feel like you are right back in high school and being peer pressured. Ugh. But he keeps right on talking. You are pretty sure you might be blushing. As he keeps yapping on about high school, you find yourself slowly, nonchalantly slipping the mask down your face until you are no longer wearing it. You feel the wind blowing against your bare mouth as you smile at your crush. You feel your insides tense up as the mask comes down.

You have just abandoned yourself. You have just broken your own rules and ignored your own boundaries to please someone else. You have made the choice to let yourself down to impress someone else. You have put your own health at risk to avoid being judged by someone else. I can almost guarantee that you will go home and stuff yourself with cake.

Here's one more example. You have done the research, seen firsthand examples, and concluded that you will not be getting the vaccine. From what you have learned, the vaccine poses more of a risk than a benefit to you. You also have concerns about long term side effects. You don't want to give it to your kids because you fear any potential complications. You are trying to make the best, safest decision for your family. You don't care what other people do but, for you, the vaccine is a no go. Okay, got it?

Now let's say that you are in group text with some friends. Normally, the group text involves making dinner plans, sharing memes, and laughing about funny experiences. Well, low and behold, someone brings up the subject of the vaccine and starts to say that people who don't get the vaccines are selfish, insensitive, assholes. Hmmmm. You stay silent. A couple of other people chime in and concur that unvaccinated people are jerks and they are causing harm to everyone. You start feeling a little awkward, uncomfortable, and, once again, bullied. You remain silent. You do notice that you are not the only silent member, thankfully. Then the members that are ranting begin to say that they will no longer attend get togethers with unvaccinated friends. You feel the peer pressure mounting. You start second guessing your choices. Are you a bad, selfish, asshole? Are you a jerk? After thinking it over you decide that you still don't believe it's the right choice but you go and get the vaccine anyway. You feel your insides turn as they administer the injection.

You have just abandoned yourself. You have just deserted your beliefs to appease others. You haven't just changed your mind about getting the vaccine. You kept the same beliefs and got the vaccine anyway. You have put your needs and wants aside to be accepted. You have abandoned your concerns for your health to fit in. Ouch. I am going to place my bets on you stuffing down these bad feelings with some major comfort food.

Obviously, I am not taking sides either way on ANY of these issues. I am just trying to make an important point. The scenarios could be switched around and used vice versa but the general idea is the same. I wanted to use these examples here because I know that this is a current topic that everyone can relate to.

Okay, so you may be asking, "I get it. I abandoned myself. But what does that even mean?? And why does it matter?? Aren't we supposed to be talking about losing weight??" Well, let's take a look.

Essentially, every time that you break a promise to yourself, or you do something that doesn't feel right to you, or you say yes when you really mean no, your body interprets it just as if someone else has done it to you. In other words, your body really knows no difference between you breaking your own promise or your boyfriend breaking a promise to you.

In either scenario, your body feels let down, rejected, and unworthy. Yikes! This is why abandoning yourself is such a no-no. This is why taking care of ourselves is SO important. When you abandon yourself, you may not be aware of it on a conscious level, but your body really does feel wounded, uncared for, and not worth a darn. And, as you can imagine, this will surely lead to some late-night snacking sessions to soothe the pain.

On the other hand, when we stand by our beliefs and keep our promises to ourselves, we are able to trust ourselves and we FEEL GOOD. It's like we are telling ourselves, "girl, I've got your back. You can count on me." We are basically our own ride-or-die. How awesome is that?

Does any of this sound familiar? How could you possibly start working on trusting yourself more? What if you start out by just working on noticing when you may be abandoning yourself? Try and catch yourself when you say yes but really want to say no. Start taking note of the times when you put your needs aside to cater to the needs of others.

Let me give you a few examples of what abandoning yourself can look like. That way you can spot it from a mile away and start to take notice when you are doing this. Here are a few possibilities:

1. You agree to pick up an extra work shift when you really don't want to and already feel overworked.
2. You don't let your boyfriend know that you are upset by something because you don't want to "cause trouble".
3. You don't speak up when your doctor suggests a treatment that you are really uncomfortable with and don't want.
4. You hit the snooze button a million times and skip the gym even though you really wanted to go to this new class and you promised yourself you would try it just once to see if you like it.
5. You say yes to a dinner party invite even though you are exhausted and want nothing more than to curl up in bed and read a good book.
6. You keep putting off filling out that college application because the idea of going back to school at your age is scary. You put it off until you have missed the deadline and it's too late.

7. You spend way more money than you are comfortable with on stuff that you don't really want or need.
8. You don't speak up when your boss piles way more than your share of work on you.
9. You don't leave toxic relationships.
10. You tolerate bad behavior from others.

Does any of this sound familiar to you? It all sounds very familiar to me. In fact, it was easy for me to come up with this list of examples because these are all experiences from my own life. These are all ways that I have abandoned myself before.

Once you have started noticing these things, then you can really start working on making changes. Maybe by trying to be better about enforcing your boundaries. Maybe by following through when you say you are going to do something. Maybe keeping your promises to yourself. I know, this crap is hard. It really is. I am still working on it every single day. Phew.

Hold on! Before we wrap this chapter up, I want to discuss one more thing that you may be telling your body. This one's a doozy and it has been a struggle for me for, what feels like, FOREVER. What is it? It's the feeling of being "too much." Have you ever felt this way? Have you ever felt like your body, your ideas, your personality, your feelings were just "too much"? Lord knows I have.

Let me give you a few examples of what feeling like "too much" might look like. This is a concept that I really want to drive home because feeling like "too much" in ANY way will, most likely, result in too many cookies, which will result in too many pounds on the scale. Ugh.

A few years ago, I was working on starting up a small business with a good friend of mine. We were both super excited and the creative juices were flowing. However, there was a nagging suspicion in the back of my mind that I was a little MORE excited than she was. I was a little MORE gung-ho than she was. I was a little MORE present than she was. There were a few conversations where I could read between the lines and see that my enthusiasm trumped hers. I didn't know it at the time, but she had other things going on in her life that also required her attention and commitment.

Well, over time, I started noticing that I was, ever so slightly, holding back my enthusiasm. I didn't want to seem too enthusiastic. I didn't want to seem too gung-ho. I was intentionally quelling my excitement because I didn't want to turn her off. I wanted this business to work so badly that

I was willing to mold myself into who I thought I needed to be to not run my business partner off. I started being less of me to avoid being TOO MUCH to her. Oh my. Not good. I was literally embarrassed that I was enthusiastic, excited, and fully committed to this new business. So, I stuffed down (ugh!) those feelings and acted cool and like it was all no big deal. I acted like I was the same level of excited, enthusiastic, and committed as she was. I told myself that I was too much. Ouch.

Can you see the danger in this? In reality, me feeling like "too much" was actually just a sign of a mismatched business pairing. It was really just a matter of two people who were in different places in life. But I took it personally and internalized it as I was "too much." My feelings were too big. My enthusiasm was too much. And what did I do with my feelings? Stuffed them down. With what? You guessed it. Food.

Here's another example. Shortly after divorcing, I dated this one guy. Well, so many things about this relationship were wrong but that's a whole different story. Long story short, he was the dating around, "busy," unavailable type and I was the newly-divorced, emotional mess, clingy type. Cringe. Anyway, he liked to go M.I.A. for days and I didn't like that so much. He was fine with having sporadic, unpredictable, no rhyme or reason contact and that ground my gears like nothing else. Needless to say, it was a disastrous "relationship."

So, as you can imagine, this entire experience left me feeling like "too much." My feelings were too strong. I wanted too much contact. I wanted more. Oof. I felt like a big, giant pile of "too much." So, what did I do? Well, if he didn't call, I made it better with cookies. If he didn't text, I dulled the pain with pizza. If he didn't show up, I treated myself to donuts. Once again, this really just boiled down to a terribly mismatched pairing, but I took it personally. And, yes, admittedly I was a post-divorce stage-five clinger at that time, but...

Anyhow, are there any areas of your life where you feel like you are "too much"? Any areas where you feel like your feelings are too big? Any areas where you feel the need to quell your enthusiasm or hide your excitement to please someone else? Any areas where you feel guilty (ugh!!!) for being "too much"?

One area this may be showing up is in your hopes and dreams. Do you secretly daydream about starting your own business? Have you always wanted to take skydiving lessons? Are you 65 years old and still dream of swimming across the Atlantic? No matter what your hopes and dreams are, you may have been told at some point that they are too much or too big. It may have been society as a whole that told you this. Or it may have been your mother. No matter where this feeling has come from, at some point in your life, you may have been led to believe that your dreams are just too darn big. "Why would a girl like you want to go skydiving?" "Don't you know that 65-year-olds don't swim across the Atlantic?" "You don't know anything about starting businesses!"

And let's look at this concept from a broader perspective. What if there were no big dreamers in this world? What if everyone stifled their wishes to please others? What if everyone dismissed their true feelings to fit in? What if everyone abandoned their hopes and dreams to fit into society? Would we have ever invented airplanes? Would we have ever reached the moon? Would we have ever discovered peanut butter and jelly sandwiches?

Also, feeling like "too much" can overflow into all areas of your life. Feeling like you are too much to put up with. Feeling like you have too many feelings. Feeling like you are too much to fit into that cute dress. Feeling like you are too big to take those scuba lessons you are dying to take. Feeling like you are too much to fit into the airplane seat. Feeling like your dream of becoming a writer at the age of sixty is too much. Feeling like your dream of living in that beautiful mansion one day is too far-fetched. You get the point. Feeling like "too much" has got to stop. I mean, what if Neil Armstrong had listened when that well-meaning friend of his had told him that the idea of walking on the moon was just downright CRAZY?

I want to tell you this right now and I am begging you to listen. You are never "too much." Never! If you ever feel like you are too much around another person, then that is not the right person for you. Or the timing is not right. Or something else is off. My point is, you are NOT too much. Please remember that. Even when you are a post-divorce, wishy-washy, emotional wreck, stage-five clinger.

Okay, let's review. We have concluded that, when we diet and binge, we are telling our bodies that we are guilty, untrustworthy, and deserving of punishment. We are also, most likely, sending strong signals to our bodies that they are unlovable, unacceptable, bad, and something to be ashamed of. We might be screaming at our bodies that they are too damn much! Ouch. This is really sad. And, since it seems undeniable that our thoughts influence our eating habits, it seems it would be a safe assumption to say that we HAVE to change these thoughts. So, let's look at a new way of thinking.

Picture a world in which you didn't obsess about food. I know, seems impossible. But stay with me here. Picture a world in which you trusted yourself to make healthy food choices and you ate intuitively. Picture a world in which you ate until satisfied and then stopped. If this was how you ate, what kind of thoughts do you think you would be thinking? What kind of beliefs about your body do you think you would hold? Let's take a look.

I would imagine that a person who ate healthily, intuitively, and without obsession would feel free, self-compassionate, and worthy of nourishment. I imagine that they would feel nurtured. I imagine this person would trust themselves to make choices that were beneficial to their well-being. I imagine this person would not be interested in punishing themselves. I imagine this person would not want to beat themselves up or hurt themselves. I imagine this person would have healthy amounts of self-esteem, self-compassion, and self-love.

Bingo. This is where the magic lies. Self-love. Self-esteem. Self-compassion. If we can master or, at least, work on increasing these then we are on our way to food freedom.

Let me give you a quick example of how these might be helpful. Consider self-compassion. Okay, you may be thinking, *what in the flip does that have to do with losing weight??* Well, think about this. Let's say you have had a really rough day and you are exhausted and feeling depleted. Maybe your boss screamed at you. Maybe your kids were swinging from the chandelier all day. Maybe you tripped and fell right in front of your crush. Whatever the reason, you are feeling DONE. The very last thing you are worried about is drumming up the willpower to avoid the chocolate chip cookies in the pantry. So, you pull up a chair and stuff yourself until you feel sick. Now what?

Well, if you are super low on self-compassion you will, most likely instantly begin beating yourself up. You will probably start telling yourself what a stupid, fat, lazy, worthless loser you are. You will, undoubtedly, conclude that the only remedy for this unacceptable behavior is to start a new crash diet in the morning and starve yourself for the next few days. You will also, most assuredly, feel it's necessary to beat yourself up and feel like a horrible person for at least the next three days.

Sound about right? Can you see how lacking self-compassion can fuel the never-ending, vicious diet/binge/starve cycle?

Let's consider the opposite scenario. Imagine if you practiced self-compassion in this moment. Okay, so you had the horrible day and you stuffed yourself with the cookies. If you can feel some compassion towards yourself, you may, instead, think to yourself, *ugh, I feel like crap. But, jeez, I had the worst day! I probably shouldn't have stuffed myself with those cookies but oh freaking well. I was seriously hurting and needed some comfort! I did it and it's over and tomorrow I will get back on track. Phew. What a day!*

Can you see how different this can be? No beating yourself up. No starting crazy crash diets that, inevitably, end in binging. No feeling like crap for days. And you know what the exciting part is? This is totally possible! I am serious! We just need to do a little work on increasing our self-compassion, self-love, and self-esteem. We can do this.

So, what do you think you are telling your body? Are you telling it that it's worthy of love and nourishment? Or are you telling it that it deserves to be abused and beaten up? Are you having compassion with it? Or are you telling it that it is being held to impossible standards?

Here is what I promise you. A long term, healthy, trim, happy body is never achieved through harsh treatment, punishment, starvation, or neglect. The body you are truly longing for, one that's life-long healthy, vibrant, fulfilled, happy, trim, and feels good, will come from love, compassion, acceptance, caring, and worthiness. It really is the only way.

Okay, so now that we have looked at what might be going on in these amazing bodies of ours, let's start working on what we can do to start losing the darn weight. In the next chapters, I am going to lay out the exact things that I have done that have led to easy, sustainable, uncomplicated, loving weight loss.

Here's the thing. It's all or nothing time. In order to see results, you really have to go all in on all of the steps. You have to really work at grasping the concepts and thinking really hard about how they apply to you. You have to do the work. And you absolutely can do this!

Let's go.

Chapter 4: *Namaste*

Several years ago I decided I was going to start meditating. I wanted to be that zen-like goddess person who always seems chill and laid back without a care in the world. And I wanted to wear the cute, little yoga clothes and smell like essential oils. I assumed that if I started meditating, all those things would fall into place. Right?

I Imagined I would suddenly be transformed into this calm, centered person who lives in joy and happiness twenty-four hours a day, seven days a week. I imagined that I would blissfully float about my day without a care in the world. I imagined that all my problems would magically disappear. Well, much to my surprise, that's not how it went.

I downloaded this app onto my phone that I had heard about. It included a fifty-day course on learning to meditate. Each day was a different meditation and each one lasted about ten minutes.

I did all the things I thought I was supposed to do to prepare. I set up my home office to be a little meditation room. I tested out about two hundred different sitting positions. I tried sitting on the floor cross-legged. I tried sitting in a chair against the wall. I tried just about every possibility I could think of.

Then I experimented with the lights. Should the lights be on or off? Should the curtains be closed, open, or partially open and partially closed? I also went through lots and lots of internal debate over whether or not I should diffuse essential oils. If so, what scent? Jeez.

Anyway, after all this crazy preparation, the day came when I was "ready" to start meditating. So, I sat for the intended ten minutes with my headphones on and listened to the speaker's gentle voice guide me through my first meditation. Okay, that wasn't so bad. Admittedly, it is kind of hard to sit still for ten straight minutes when you aren't used to it, but it wasn't pure misery either. It was easy enough that I returned the next day.

Day two I was a little more antsy. I was fidgety and, honestly, kept opening my eyes and glancing at my phone to see how much time was left. It felt a little more difficult this time. I mean, I had things to do for goodness sake!

Day three was much like day two. I was antsy again. I was itching to abandon the whole idea of meditation. I mean, this doesn't seem to be doing anything!

On day four I resolved to do my best to be more serious about it and try to be "present." I made myself sit still even when the unbearable urge to fidget would come. I did my best to focus on my breathing.

The days went on like this. Some days I was antsy and some days I was beginning to be able to survive the entire ten minutes without fidgeting. The first couple of weeks of my meditation practice were weird. I noticed that I was feeling angry frequently. I was a little more snappy with my kids. But I was aware of it. I noticed the feelings. Hmmm.

A few weeks into my meditation practice, things started changing. I was no longer angry and snappy. I was starting to feel what I can only explain as "slow." Huh? I know, weird, right? What on Earth do I mean by "slow"?

Well, the only way that I can describe it is to say that I started to have the sensation that time was slowing down. In a good way. And my reactions were slowing down. In a good way. I was becoming less reactive to everything. I was not joy-filled 24/7. I was not suddenly the happiest person on Earth. I was not suddenly Mary Poppins. Instead, I was less reactive.

Okay, so why does this even remotely matter to you? Well, let me explain all the amazing benefits of being less reactive a little further.

The very first thing I noticed about myself was that I was less snappy with my kids. That, in and of itself, is a super awesome thing! Next up, I started noticing that I was more laid back around people that typically irritated me. For instance, prior to starting my meditation practice, if one of my coworkers said something that irked me and I just knew that they were wrong, I would have been instantly irritated and felt the need to argue until I proved I was right and they were wrong. Oof. After I had been meditating for a few months, I started noticing that, if someone said something I disagreed with, I would not even feel the urge to argue the point. I would be more likely to think to myself, *oh well, I am pretty sure they are wrong but I literally don't even care. They can have their view and I'll have mine. It's whatever.*

Okay, first of all, this felt like I clearly had been drinking some strange tea to even feel this way. I mean, where were my reactions? Where were my typical feisty, angry, get-all-worked-up-about-it tendencies?? Where did they go? And what were these new, chill, laid back, unruffled feathers that I was sporting? This felt like a whole new world. A "slow" world. A world in which I was able to slow time down and process what was happening in the moment, process my reactions, and stay present in the moment. I no longer felt bombshells of reactivity going off inside me. They had just disappeared!

What was crazy was that, as time went on and I continued my meditation practice, I only got better and better with my "slowness" and non-reactivity. It has now gotten to the point where you can stand in front of me and scream at me telling me that the grass is purple and I will just say, "okay, whatever. It sure is." I feel almost zero need to argue or prove any different. Well, I should emphasize "almost," because I am still a human being and there are definitely still a few things that may sneak up and ruffle my feathers. Sheesh. But, for the most part, I have tamed my feisty ways. Which, to me, seems monumental.

So, what on Earth am I telling you all of this for and can we already get to the freaking weight loss info?? I know, I know. But, I promise you, this IS part of the weight loss info.

Like I said just a minute ago, meditation has led me to feel more slowed down, less reactive, and more able to be in the present moment. So how do you think these could be valuable tools in the weight loss toolbox? Well, let's look at a few examples. I am going to tell you about a few experiences I have had where I noticed that my ability to make healthy food choices could be directly attributed to meditation.

A few weeks ago, I had a crazy hectic weekend that involved exhaustion, anxiety, and irritation. Typically, in this scenario, I would feel like a frazzled hot mess and I would feel determined that the only possible thing to make myself feel better would be warm, sticky, sweet donuts. YUM. I was absolutely sure that I HAD to have donuts and nothing else would suffice. I know you know the feeling. It's like an obsession comes over you that you can't control, and you can't stop until you complete your mission. It feels all-consuming, uncontrollable, and unstoppable. It makes you feel like a prisoner of your own mind. Like a drug addict who NEEDS a fix. Literally. It feels horrible.

Anyway, in this instance, I had a different experience. Yes, I had the crappy weekend. Yes, I had the extreme urge for donuts. But here's where things were different. I set out in my car telling myself that I could go get the donuts. As I drove in the general direction of the donut shop, I did some deep breathing and thought about what was going on inside of me.

Was I really hungry? Deep breath in and out. Did I really want donuts or was I desperately seeking something to soothe my nerves? Deep breath in and out. Was I really willing to put my body through the torturous aftermath of a donut binge for just a minute of pleasure? Deep breath in and out. Didn't I remember just how absolutely disgusting and nauseous I would feel immediately following a binge? Deep breath in and out. Didn't I remember the horrible feelings of hatred I would have for myself if I caved and ate the donuts? Deep breath in and out. What would happen if I chose to, instead, drive around for just a minute longer and think about these things? Deep breath in and out. What if I acknowledged that, in this moment, I am actually having a crisis and, given a little bit of time and clarity, this crisis will pass? Deep breath in and out. What if I consider that what's really going on is that I just feel like crying and I could use a giant hug and some love? Deep breath in and out. What if I breathe for a minute and actually feel the pain I am feeling and let myself cry? Deep breath in and out. What if I choose to hear my body's cry for attention and choose to give it that attention instead of denying it and stifling it with donuts? Deep breath in and out. What if I allow myself to consider that just getting in my car alone, driving around, listening to some good music, and deep breathing can feel almost as soothing as a quick fix of donuts? Deep breath in and out. What if I drive a little longer and see if I can get the donut urge to pass? Deep breath in and out. What if I give myself complete permission to have the donuts but vow that I will try, for at least the next 15-20 minutes to sooth myself instead?

Deep breath in and out. Just drive. Deep breath in and out. Just listen to that song. Deep breath in and out. Just drive. Listen. Soothe. What if I allow myself to go get a warm, soothing tea for now? Deep breath in and out. If the tea doesn't work, I can still get the donuts. Deep breath in and out. Coffee shop here I come for a warm, chamomile tea with just a splash of honey to treat myself. Deep breath in and out. Warm tea with honey. Driving all alone with absolutely no destination in mind. Deep breath in and out. Favorite music on the radio. Deep breath in and out. Windows rolled down. Deep breath in and out. Favorite song turned up loud. Deep breath in and out. The crisis has passed. No donuts needed today.

What has just happened? Well, I have actively, purposefully, calmly soothed myself. I stayed in the present moment and talked my way through a crisis. I gave myself permission to get the donuts if I wanted to, but I was able to slow my thinking and processes down enough to be able to mentally work my way through this crisis. I was able to acknowledge that what was really happening was that I was in pain and wanting comfort. I was able to be in the moment and see the binge for what it was and talk my way out of it. This, my friends, is no less than a miracle. Seriously. A flipping miracle.

The only thing I can attribute this to is meditation. The ability to slow myself down, see the moment for what it is (a crisis), and breathe my way through it is 100% a result of meditation.

I need to point out here that an important side note would be that I am still not 100% successful with this. I still have my moments when I cave and get the donuts. I am not perfect. BUT, my theory is that if I can be successful more times than I am unsuccessful, then I win.

Let's say that you currently binge on donuts four times a week. What if meditation could cut that down to two times a week? Wouldn't you consider that a win? I think so. And what if you could cut it down to once a week? Sure seems like a win to me.

Before I started meditating, there was absolutely nothing standing between me and the donut shop. It was pedal to the metal the whole way there. My brain felt frazzled, I was a ball of nerves, and the ONLY thing that would make it all better was a box of chocolate-covered, glazed deliciousness. God forbid you get in my way during one of these episodes. Yikes. My point is, in those instances I would have looked at you like you were an alien if you suggested I try soothing myself instead of gorging myself with sugar. It just didn't seem possible.

Let's say that you do cave and eat the donuts. Because we ALL do sometimes. One thing I have noticed since I began meditating is that, if I do end up eating the donuts, I am able to be "slower" about it. It doesn't always feel like a desperate, hurried, frazzled emergency. Yes, I obviously still am urgently wanting the donuts but the whole process seems a bit more slowed down and a bit more manageable. It doesn't feel quite as emergent.

So what does this mean? Well, it often means that if I cave and get the donuts, I can sometimes soothe myself with just two donuts instead of three. I can sometimes end the binge without eating an entire dozen. I can quell my thirst for soothing with fewer hits of my drug of choice.

Let's look at the overall effects of meditation on my eating habits. My experience has been that, due to the slowing down and less reactive results of meditation, I have been able to reduce the frequency and potency of my binges. They happen less often and, when they do happen, they are not as bad as before.

A couple of years ago, a binge might include a frantic trip to the fast-food place to get a double cheeseburger and fries, followed by a trip to the donut store to get something sweet to follow up with. And I would consume it all. I would be momentarily soothed but then spend days kicking myself and hating myself and feeling sick.

Now, if I feel a donut binge coming on, even if I give in and let myself get the donuts, I can eat two or three and be satisfied and move on. I don't need to do the whole thing of getting pizza and cheeseburgers and fries and donuts and cookies and stuffing myself for HOURS. And, in turn, I don't need to do the whole punishment thing for the next few days. I can quickly move on and get back into my healthy eating without beating myself up. Doesn't that sound so much better??

I am such a big believer in the power of meditation that I wanted it to be one of the very first things you incorporate into your life. So, okay great, you are probably wondering what I want you to do and how long for and what are all the details. Well, it's super simple. You can start really small.

I want you to commit to five minutes a day to begin with. Obviously, if you are a seasoned meditator, then you can continue on where you are. But, if you are new to meditation, start with five minutes. The only requirements are that you find a somewhat quiet and private space where you won't be interrupted. You can sit on the floor. You can sit in a chair. You can stand on your head. It doesn't matter. As long as you are comfortable and can stay somewhat still in your position for at least five minutes. You can put a little timer on your phone or, better yet, if you have the ability, you can download one of the many meditation apps that are available. Just do your best to sit quietly and calm your mind and focus on your breathing.

I am by no means a meditation teacher so, honestly, I could probably screw you up by trying to instruct you. Yikes! So, I would recommend getting one of the meditation apps or watching some YouTube videos or something like that. I started out with (and highly recommend!) the Waking Up app by Sam Harris. It has a fifty day meditation course that seriously changed my life. But, if that one is not available to you, I am sure there are a gazillion more.

I just can't express enough how valuable meditation can be to your WHOLE life. And, with a little luck and commitment to practice, it just might have you saying, "no, thanks. I'm good" to that fourth donut. And that, my friends, is priceless.

So, break out those zen-like vibes and get your meditation on.

Namaste.

Chapter 5: *Ditching the Diet Mindset*

Wait, what? Stop dieting? How on Earth will I ever lose weight??? Okay, hear me out. I want you to stop for one second and consider something. How has dieting worked out for you?

I mean this with every bit of love in my heart and seriously no snarkiness. I honestly want you to sit and think for one second about how dieting has worked out for you in the past.

If you are anything like me, you have struggled with this for years and lost and gained countless pounds. You may have tried every diet under the sun. Some may have worked for a time. Some may not have. Regardless, if you are reading this, I would presume that your eating habits and/or weight leave something to be desired.

I can honestly sit here right now and say, with 1000% accuracy and honesty, that no diet has ever worked for me. I mean, yes, I have lost weight on diets before. Yes, I have dropped a few quick pounds here and there. And, yes, I have even lost significant amounts of weight by dieting. That's not what I am talking about when I say that no diet has ever worked for me. What I mean is, no diet has ever transformed my lifestyle and turned me into a thin, happy, and healthy goddess for life. No diet has ever STUCK.

Every single attempt at dieting has resulted in the same (more or less) outcome. I get all geared up for the diet. I stick to the diet for a few weeks (give or take) and lose some weight. And then I fall off the wagon and start binging. And all the weight comes creeping back. And maybe even more weight.

I have decided that, for me, dieting is really just an attempt at control and punishment over my body. When I am feeling fat, unattractive, and unhealthy, I feel an overwhelming urge to take control of the situation. It's like looking at a sink full of dirty dishes. I feel an uncontrollable need to clean it up. I know, WEIRD. But I have come to be aware of this same phenomenon in my eating habits. Let me explain.

It all starts with me feeling absolutely horrible about the state of my body. I feel like I absolutely need to take control of the situation or else I will go bonkers. So, I plan out a diet (most likely whatever the current, popular diet is) and get to work taking control of the situation. I start the diet and stick to it for however long. I feel good and feel like I am in control of the situation and finally have a handle on things.

But, after however long, I start feeling exhausted by having to be so in control. I start feeling worn down by the rigidity. I start feeling sick of the control! And I start having an overwhelming need to eat what and when I want. I want to be free!

So, I think to myself, *screw this! I am going to eat whatever the heck I want and I am NOT going to feel bad about it! I won't be controlled!* So, I quit the diet.

And I instantly feel this beautiful feeling of freedom. It washes over me and I almost feel euphoric. I am free!! This freedom feels good for a while. I eat what the heck I want and when the heck I want and don't feel controlled.

Then, as to be expected, some pounds start creeping back and I start feeling fat and unhealthy again. I start feeling completely out of control again. I start feeling like I need to take control of the situation again and the whole cycle starts all over. Ugh.

So, in my opinion (which is by no means an expert opinion!), dieting is really just a fancy cover up for controlling. And I don't like to be controlled! So, it makes sense to me that we have to just completely drop the dieting mindset. We have to see it, acknowledge it, and overcome it. We have to be free from it.

What if, instead, we trained our minds to think long term and to think of food as nourishment? What if we could get to the place where we calmly make our food choices instead of being in the frantic, diet mindset of desperation? What if we could meditate and deep breathe ourselves through anxious thoughts instead of resorting to eating that box of donuts? Yes, please!

I am a firm believer that it makes no difference what "diet" you are on. What matters is if you consider it a diet. If you consider your current eating situation and it even remotely brings you a feeling of rigidity and "dieting," then it has to go. It's not going to work.

As absolutely scary as it feels, we have to stop dieting. We have to completely stop feeling deprived. We have to stop feeling starved. We have to stop feeling controlled. We have to start slowing our minds down and trusting ourselves.

In the past, when I thought of not being on some form of a diet, I thought to myself, *Oh God no, I could never just be set free to eat whatever I want! I might eat the entire grocery store! I can't be trusted! I might start grazing and never stop!* I didn't trust myself. I didn't believe in myself. I thought that, if left to my own devices, I would go on a food rampage and blow up like a balloon and probably pop. Yikes. I had literally zero trust in myself. And with good reason. I mean, my history with food wasn't really something to be proud of. I felt like if I didn't have strict control over myself and my eating, I may spiral out of control and never be able to recover. And that's freaking scary.

So, all of that being said, I 100% understand how flipping scary it can be to consider giving up dieting. I mean, I may as well suggest that you sell your house and move to Jupiter (the planet, not Florida). It sounds CRAZY! But I believe in the power of quitting dieting. And I believe that diets don't work long term. And, I mean, do you really want to be dieting and miserable for the rest of your life? I, for one, do not.

Obviously, there are going to be certain situations and reasons that some people do need to be on certain diets. If you have a disease or condition or allergy or whatever that makes it imperative that you follow a certain diet, then, by all means, please do! Always follow your doctor's guidance.

But I still believe that, no matter what your circumstances are, what we are shooting for here is the loss of the diet mindset. If you know you cannot eat gluten but you still FEEL like you are not on a diet, then that's perfect! If you cannot eat sugar but you still FEEL like you eat abundantly and you don't feel starved or deprived, then you are winning! We are shooting for the feeling of healthy, abundant, nutritious, free eating. We are trying to do away with all deprived, controlled, starved, scarce eating.

Another problem that I have with dieting is that I don't think that any one diet necessarily fits every single person all the time. I think that all of our bodies are different, and we each require individual tweaks and accommodations. And, like I just said, it's always best to check with your doctor about this. Anyhow, the point is that we can have individual needs that don't apply to others and vice versa. And, if we are being completely honest here, most of the time I don't believe the weight we are carrying is even about the food. I mean, yeah, obviously it's about the food and the calories, but it's also about other things, like our inner world and our stress levels and our beliefs.

So, I am here today to free you. You are officially granted permission to step off the diet train and take a seat in the classroom of healthy, nourishing, free eating. Hallelujah! It's time to bid sayonara to the desperation, starvation, and punishment. It's lights out for rigid, miserable, unhealthy, controlling, frantic behavior.

Instead, we are saying hello to healthy, abundant nourishment. We are saying welcome to freedom, deliciousness, and peace. I promise you that, if you incorporate the steps in this book, you can feel true food freedom and ditch the relentless obsession of dieting.

So, starting today, say goodbye to dieting and say hello to health and happiness.

Chapter 6: What's Weighing You Down?

After I got divorced, I moved three times over the course of just a few years. Needless to say, that's a lot of packing and unpacking. A lot of baggage. For a solid few years, a decent amount of my belongings remained in boxes. I would have kept the boxes limited to a spare bedroom but, unfortunately, two of the houses we lived in didn't have enough bedrooms to use one as a spare. So the boxes were often stuffed in corners, stacked in full closets, and packed under beds and tables. But no matter how hard I tried to keep them out of sight, they were there. And, honestly, I knew that two of the houses we were living in would not be permanent, so why unpack? So, our baggage stayed out in plain sight.

How is this relevant to losing weight? Well, one of the points that I want to make in this chapter is that the environment you are living in is often a direct reflection of what's going on inside of you. I was newly divorced during this time in my life. So, it would not be a giant leap to say that I was carrying around a lot of baggage; literally AND figuratively. For those first few years following divorce, you probably could have walked into my home and made a pretty accurate guess about what was going on inside of me.

Having boxes randomly scattered around my house was not the only issue during this time. I was also, at any given time, working three or four jobs while also doing my best to be a full-time mom. It's pretty safe to say that on most days my house did not look like the pages of a magazine. I tried my very hardest to keep it clean and organized but there was only so much I could do. The grass was often uncut. There was often a stack of mail and papers on the kitchen counter.

There were often dirty dishes in the sink. And the last thing I had the money for was a housekeeper. If I didn't do it, it wasn't getting done.

Did I mention the stack of mail unopened on the kitchen counter? Another issue lurking during this season of my life was the state of my finances. I was broke. Really broke. I was living paycheck to paycheck and most weeks the paychecks didn't even cover all my expenses. I went through a whole period of making really bad decisions regarding money and digging myself deeper and deeper into debt. It wasn't pretty.

And when you are living paycheck to paycheck, some things around the house have to take a back seat to more important things like eating and gas. So this meant that if the dishwasher was broken, it was time to put on some gloves and get to hand washing. If the lawn mower was broken, then put on some boots because you will be walking through three-foot-high grass. And if you accidentally put a hole in the wall while moving furniture? Well then you can just hang a picture right over that hole because there is no money in the bank for a repairman.

Another aspect of this whole time in my life was the fact that since I was a newly single mom, it meant that I was the only adult in my house.

Therefore, everything was my responsibility. The yard work, the repairs, the upkeep, the expenses, and everything else. You could say I had the weight of the world on me. Literally.

Stop and think about this for one second. If you are so swamped in your life right now, is it likely that you have any time to practice self-care? I doubt it. If you are carrying the weight of the world on your shoulders, does that leave any room for thinking of yourself? Probably not. If your house is filled with unpacked boxes, or your grass is uncut, or the stack of bills on your kitchen counter is four feet high, do you really believe that you are in the right mental place to love and care for your body? I know I wasn't.

I want you to look around at your environment. How are you living? What does your life look like? Are you stepping over piles of laundry to get to the bathroom? Is your dining table used for paperwork storage instead of eating? Do you look at your house and think to yourself, *my house looks an awful lot like an episode of Hoarders!* Ugh. I know, I totally get it. I have been there. I have done the hoarding. I have made my way from my front door to my car by walking through tall grass and weeds. I felt like I was going to absolutely fall over and die from embarrassment about what the neighbors must think about my unkempt yard. I had that stack of unpaid bills sit on the counter ignored for months. I had dirty dishes sit in the sink while my kids and I ate off of paper plates because that's so much freaking easier. I get it.

So. The very first step in this process is just assessing your situation. No shame here. Just take an honest look around you and take note of what you see.

Your house. Is it clean? Is it a hot mess? Is it cluttered? Is it neat and tidy? What is it? The first step in this process is to focus your energy on improving the vibe of your environment. I know you are probably extremely busy. I know time is hard to come by. And I know that the last thing you may want to do on a Saturday is clean your house. But I want you to. If you need to, start small. Clean one bathroom. Clean out one junk drawer in your kitchen. Organize your coat closet. It doesn't matter how small you start, just start! I seriously promise you that tidying up will make you feel good in your bones! Even though it sounds bonkers, there is tremendous power in the simple act of cleaning your home. Visualize your house as your body. Do you want it cluttered, stuffed, and embarrassing? Or would you prefer to have it uncluttered, tidy, and taken care of?

Now that you have started tidying up and organizing your house, what on Earth do you do with all this stuff? There's only so much closet and attic space a person can have. And, in my opinion, clutter is like fingernails on a chalkboard. Clutter causes my anxiety to skyrocket and is guaranteed to make me want to eat an entire pizza and finish it off with a sleeve of Oreos.

So, what's the remedy here? Give it away! Seriously! Give the crap away. I used to be super sentimental about all of my "things." That t-shirt from 1995 that I never even wore but it reminded me of college? How on Earth could I ever get rid of that? That picture frame that doesn't match anything in my house and I hate the look of it, but it was only $1? I can't tell it goodbye! That ice cream maker that I paid a fortune for eight years ago and only used once? Why on Earth would I want to give that away?

Well, guess what? We are saying goodbye! As hard as it may feel to part ways, the feeling of having an uncluttered and tidy house is so worth it! And, if that's not enough to make you kiss the crap goodbye, think of the people that you may help by donating your stuff. That t-shirt from 1995 just might be a perfect fit on that little boy who hasn't had a new shirt in two years. That picture frame might be exactly what that cute little grandma was looking for to put a picture of her grandkids in. And that ice cream maker might make some sweet little girl the happiest girl on Earth on Christmas morning. Now that feels good! So let's get to giving! You can pack up anything you want to give away and drop it off at Goodwill or whatever donation place your area has. And there are even some donation places that will come and pick the stuff up from your front porch. Easy peasy, lemon squeezzy! Think of it as though you are literally giving your baggage away! Here, come and take this extra weight! Literally!

Beep beep! How's your car looking these days? Has it not had a bath in two years? Are there fast-food bags stacked two feet high on the back seat? Wait, what is that I see there? Are those roaches crawling out from under your seat?? No worries, we have ALL been there. I don't care if you drive a Ford Pinto or the latest Range Rover. What I am talking about here is the condition of your car. You know that incredible feeling when you go to the car wash and vacuum your car and go through the washer and you drive away feeling like a million bucks? Let's do it! After all, your car is just another extension of your living space so it's gonna need attention too.

Okay, let's switch gears. Holy money. How tall is the stack of bills on your kitchen counter? How many times have you walked right on past it and thought to yourself, *ugh, I REALLY need to deal with that but the thought of actually doing it makes me want to stab a needle in my eye!*

I know, I have felt that exact way soooooo many times. Facing the truth about your financial situation and actually taking steps to address it can feel overwhelming, scary as hell, and, quite frankly, hopeless.

I remember days when I would walk past the stack of bills on my counter and think to myself, *I am pretty much broke so what's the point of opening those bills anyway?* Well, here's the thing. If you are in a place in your life where you are financially strapped, highly stressed about money, or fearing that the bank will foreclose on your house at any minute, you may not be in the ideal position to mentally devote to nurturing your body. You are, most likely, instead, in a place to want to punish your body. Does that make sense?

When I was at the height of my financial problems (foreclosure, near bankruptcy), there was no way that I was in the proper headspace for self-improvement and becoming healthy. I was a mess. Inside and out. The last thing I was worried about was whether or not I was getting enough protein. And I would have laughed out loud if you would have suggested I take a day off and go to the spa. I barely had the money for the gas required to drive to the spa.

So, let's see what we can do to clean this area up a little for you. Go ahead and open those bills. See if you can do anything at all to resolve any outstanding issues. Can you work out some payment plans? Can you pay off that loan? Can you make a budget? Can you call that finance company and tell them that, even though you can't afford your payment right now, your intentions are good and you want to work with them? Even if you are doing pretty well in the finances department, is there any area that could use a little attention?

What I learned from my time spent in financial despair was that taking even the smallest of steps towards working on it will make you feel a little better, a little more in control, and a little more like you are doing the right thing. Addressing the issues and working on them, even the tiniest bit, usually makes you feel a little better about yourself. And that's exactly the vibe we are shooting for in this book!

Speaking of stress. Let's take a minute and talk about this beast. I argue that you are paddling upstream if you try to lose weight while you are super stressed. Unless, of course, you are extremely stressed and not eating anything. And that's a whole different story and not what we are talking about here.

Stress and anxiety are so detrimental to our health and well-being. And they will sabotage even the hardest of efforts to get healthy. Stressful situations cause your body to increase production of the stress hormone cortisol. I won't go into too much science here, but this increase in cortisol levels is not what you want. Increases in cortisol promote fat storage and rapid weight gain. YIKES!

I don't know about you, but I am pretty much guaranteed to plow through my kitchen after having a stressful day. It happens every time. Bad day at work? I am definitely eating donuts. Stuck in traffic and late to an important event? Oh yeah, I am shoveling down the chocolate. My kid just got suspended from school? Well, it hasn't happened (yet) but I imagine I would eat ALL the desserts.

I don't think it matters what the stressful situation is or how severe it is. All that matters is that it's stress. And if you are feeling stress on a daily basis, I would imagine that your body is feeling the bad vibes. Aside from causing weight gain, it is widely known that stress is linked to other medical conditions like cardiovascular disease, inflammation, mental illness, and stroke. So, it's got to go!

Like I said earlier, after getting divorced and becoming a single mom, I was STRESSED. I was working nonstop, trying to be a good mom, and constantly freaking out about money. I also had no time for exercise. And my only comfort during this time was food. Cinnamon rolls were my best friend and they never let me down. And they made me feel soothed. Needless to say, I started rapidly packing on the pounds. It was shocking how I went from a relatively fit and healthy person to a stressed out, overweight, tired and achy person. I felt horrible.

Several years went by where I was living day in and day out in this stressed out, anxious, uncomfortable, fat life. I was miserable. But over time, my life began to calm down. My job situation became more manageable. I worked my money problems out. I started finding time for a little exercise. I got rid of toxic situations in my life. I started meditating. Overall, my life became less stressful. And that's when the weight started coming off.

Without even "trying," my body started to drop some weight when my stress decreased. It almost felt like I had been literally carrying all this stress and baggage around and when I focused on ditching the stress and baggage, my body was able to let go.

What can you let go of today? Is there an area of your life that feels like "baggage"? Is there ongoing stress in your life that needs to be kicked to the curb? Obviously, there may be some stressful situations that we just can't "fix." Maybe you have a sick child. Or maybe you are caring for a parent with dementia. Or maybe some other stressful situation that you have to live with. If that's the case, my heart seriously goes out to you and I am sending you all the good vibes and hugs in the world.

Sit down and make a list of stressful things in your life. I urge you to look at how you can fix or get rid of these situations. Again, this may require baby steps but every step counts! Since I can't tell you exactly how to fix or get rid of every stressful situation in your life, I am going to list here some possible situations that may be stress sources in your life.

Money! We just talked about getting organized in the financial department. I am such a believer in how horribly stressful money can be, so I want to list it first. I have personally been through financial despair, including my house going into foreclosure and almost having to file bankruptcy. I have never felt stress like that before. So, if you are feeling stressed about money, I urge you to see if there's any way that you can figure it out or ease your mind about it.

Here's a bit of encouragement. I believe with every ounce of my being that money problems always work themselves out. Also, as bananas as this sounds, all money problems (including foreclosure and bankruptcy!) are survivable. Really! I know, because I have survived them!

And here's a pro tip. As whacky as this sounds, in an effort to improve your finances, focus on improving your self-esteem. Really try and bump up your self-worth. This worked wonders for me! After all, what are you worth? Millions or pennies? See the correlation?

Okay, what about your job. Even if you wouldn't classify your job as toxic and you like your job, does it cause you to feel stressed too frequently? What can be done to change this?

Next up, relationships. Do any of your relationships cause you stress? Are there any changes you could make, or boundaries you could set, that would make these relationships less stressful?

Your schedule. Do you find that most of your time is spent in traffic? Do you sacrifice your exercise time when someone asks you to do something else? Do you stay up way too late at night looking at your phone? Personally, I know I seriously can go way overboard with playing on my phone if I don't stop myself. In the past I have skipped exercise class because I was tied up in a serious game of Candy Crush. Ugh.

Your environment. Again, we talked about this already but it's worth mentioning again. At the height of my stressful period, I would look out the window at the overgrown grass and overtaking weeds and I would feel STRESS. I would look at the piles of laundry and feel stress. I would see the dishes in the sink and feel stress. I would get into my dirty car to go to work and feel stress.

And here's an example of my personal experience with environmental stress. My dog is a yapper. I mean, a real yapper. I can come home from the hardest day at work and get into a warm bubble bath and take a deep breath and relax. And guess what happens then? My dog will start barking as if our house is being invaded by Martians. And it will go on for the whole darn time I am in the freaking bathtub. And it's so loud! I swear my blood pressure skyrockets.

So, after suffering through years of disrupted bubble baths, something had to change. I started leaving the back door cracked open and letting my dog play in the back yard while I take a bath. Voila! No more barking! I mean, an axe murderer may come in the open back door and kill me but I'll take my chances. What can you do today to make your environment less stressful?

Your to-do list. Does is make your blood pressure soar? Okay, this one is difficult. Why? Because it sounds like all I have done so far in this book is give you one long to-do list! So how can I rationally tell you not to stress about your to-do list. I can't. I guess what I will say here is that I urge you to focus as much as you can on the things that cause you the most stress and try your hardest not to even think about the others. Because the very last thing I intend to do here is cause you stress! Also, just remember that NOBODY ever checks off every item on their to-do list. If they do, then they are definitely not human.

Oftentimes, when I get all caught up in stressing out over little things, I suddenly remember that most of this crap really doesn't even matter. I mean, REALLY. In the end, it does not matter one freaking bit if my house is clean every day. It doesn't matter even the slightest if I checked off everything on my to-do list. Do we have electricity? Okay, we're good. Do we all have our health and our bodies intact? We are soooo good. Do we have food to eat and roofs over our heads? YES! Those are the things that matter. Everything else is just extra. And everything else doesn't deserve our stress. So, let's ditch the stress and get to living our damn lives!

Okay, here we go. We are switching gears again. Now I want to work on doing a little detoxing. No, not food or drink detox. Not alcohol or drugs detox. I mean PEOPLE detox. I mean toxic situations and bad vibes detox. I mean detox from anything that's bringing you down. It's all got to go. Like yesterday. If you haven't caught on yet, the entire point of this chapter is to say goodbye to any and every thing that may be weighing you down. And that, my friend, includes people.

I once had a person in my life who was the very definition of toxic. Critical, negative, judgmental, demeaning, manipulative, and all the bad things. Her presence just felt icky and infuriating. She was confrontational and aggressive. And given that I HATE confrontation and try to avoid it at all costs, she was not at all a good fit for me. She was the kind of person that was always stirring the pot and she always had something negative to say about someone and always wanted to gossip. Ugh.

Needless to say, this woman weighed me down. Literally. After being in her presence or having contact with her, I felt horrible. I felt sad. I felt like my nerves were frayed. Looking back, it was usually after an interaction involving her when I would binge. I would eat my feelings.

Here's how it would go. I would interact with her. I felt manipulated, cornered, dirty, and/or some other negative feeling. I was scared to speak up and create boundaries or, for some other reason, it was just not appropriate to do so. Or, more likely, I just didn't even feel like dealing with this person and, at all costs, did anything to escape engaging with her. Regardless, this left me with all of these pent-up negative emotions and feelings after every interaction with her. I never was able to speak up and say how I felt. So I ate.

And I ate a lot. I ate my feelings and I stuffed them down. I buried them with food. I ate until I didn't feel angry anymore.

Do you see the correlation here? Every time I would interact with this specific woman, I would wind up feeling wiped out, beaten up, anxiety-ridden, and gross. I couldn't speak my true feelings to her. Subsequently, I would make myself feel better by stuffing my feelings down with delicious, comforting, dopamine-releasing treats. And I would feel better. It worked every time. And I didn't even realize that that was what I was doing.

I have also realized that I have a high probability of binging when I feel shut down by someone. Recently, I made a clinical judgement about something at work using my best nursing skills. One of my coworkers came along shortly after and second guessed me, micromanaged the situation and took over. I felt completely shut down and walked over. I felt defeated. But my only option would have been to argue the point and, after feeling shut down, I didn't even care or want to. So I went home and ate cookies.

Here's the thing. There are certain people in this world who, for whatever reason, you will never be able to speak your truth to. These people are toxic to you. If you hang around people who you feel uncomfortable being your real self around, then that is NOT healthy to you. If you have an abusive or manipulative person in your life and for your own safety or peace of mind you have to keep your mouth shut and your feelings to yourself, then that person is highly toxic to you. And you will be stuffing your feelings down. Most likely with a dozen donuts and an ice cream sundae.

Another type of person that you might find yourself dealing with is the person that gets you to carry their load for them. These types of people are not necessarily "toxic" to you as those just described, but they can be just as detrimental to your self-care and weight loss. These are people that may not be negative, or aggressive, or demeaning, but they, instead, give you their needs and burdens to carry. And we often "carry" them on our hips and stomachs and butts. Ugh.

Do you have someone in your life that is always asking you to do something? Or someone that constantly needs your encouragement, emotional support, pep talks, and/or coaching? Someone that can't seem to think for themselves or accomplish anything on their own? Well, maybe it's time for you to quit carrying it ALL for them.

Maybe you could give them back a little of their baggage and let them carry it.

Toxicity in your life doesn't always just come from friends, or family, or other people in your life. How's your job? Do you bust your butt day in and day out for a boss who makes you walk on eggshells? Or do you have a job that feels like aspects of it are not in line with your core beliefs as a human being? Or maybe you are a stay-at-home mom and you absolutely hate it and would give anything to go back to work. Whatever your situation is with your day to day "job," if it's bringing you down then something needs to change.

Several years ago I was working as a nurse for a certain company full time. The actual patient care part of the job was enjoyable to me. It was the other aspects that were completely toxic. The other nurses and I were consistently pushed to work overtime. The amount of paperwork that was expected kept increasing. And we would regularly receive threatening texts from our boss making it sound like we would be fired if we didn't comply.

Needless to say, this job was stressful. My anxiety level was sky high. I was angry constantly but felt like I couldn't speak up for fear of losing my job.

I was a newly single mom at the time so losing my job was not an option. I kept my mouth shut. And this is when I started packing on the pounds. I would spend my days working myself to exhaustion, feeling manipulated and belittled and threatened, and then go home angry and starving. This was a recipe for disaster. In the course of a year I gained thirty pounds. Yikes.

At the other end of the spectrum, lacking a job or other creative outlet can be a problem too. When my kids were little, I was a stay-at-home mom for several years. I wouldn't trade that time for anything in the world. I loved being there for my kids and I would never regret that. I was there for every single milestone in their adorable little lives.

BUT, I often found myself going stir crazy. I often found myself aching for something to "work" on, or a project or a job to do. I longed for adult interaction and having coworkers to shoot the breeze with, and I even missed getting dressed for work and having a schedule. There were days when I would have given anything to be sitting in a cold conference room participating in a boring work meeting.

Suffice it to say, I was bored. During the long afternoon stretches when my babies would be napping, I sometimes felt like a caged animal pacing the hallway. So, what did I do? I baked cookies! I baked pies! I baked cupcakes! Then what did I do? I ate them! Well, not all of them. But I definitely ate my share. Sweet treats became the excitement of my life. I know, sad. Clearly, I was bored and looking for some excitement and a creative outlet. And fresh baked goods were the answer.

Looking back, I probably should have put a little more effort into finding creative outlets for myself. I should have dropped some of the mommy guilt and gotten a darn babysitter more often so that I could get out of the house. There were, on occasion, long stretches of time (like weeks) when I didn't have a single hour to myself that I could remember. That, without a doubt, can become a potentially toxic problem.

Speaking of toxic, I have heard of studies stating that there is some evidence that fat ITSELF is toxic. I have heard that the cells that fat is comprised of can be toxic to your body. I have read several studies that say that inside fat are stored toxins from the environment, the foods you eat, and other things you put into your body. Yikes! So how could it possibly be a stretch to say that hanging around and absorbing toxic situations and people could be related to actual fat on your body? It makes sense to me. I mean, if you're going to be consistently exposed to toxic stuff, it's got to be stored somewhere, right?

Nevertheless, I have found that when my life is mostly free from toxic people and situations, I feel less inclined to binge. I feel less of the anxiety that so often leads to me stuffing myself. I feel, by nature, detoxed.

Do you have toxic people or situations in your life? What can you do today to change that? Are there boundaries you can set with certain people, or people that you need to just completely cut out? Can you start working on your resume to get yourself out of the toxic jail you may be in? Are there some tweaks in your daily routine that you can make that will lighten your load that you carry?

First, let's sit down and make a list of any people or situations that feel toxic. As always, the first step is to identify the problem. Some people and situations may immediately come to mind and some others may require a little contemplation.

What does toxic feel like? Well, for me, toxic people and situations always leave me feeling icky. You may possibly feel some combination of bullied, used, depressed, angry, "bad," exhausted, manipulated, stuck, frustrated, disrespected, dirty, judged, and/or unhappy. Do you have a person or people in your life that, after interacting with them, you feel any of these ways? Do you have a job or other situation that leaves you feeling like this?

Now, obviously, there may be, from time to time, days when our jobs or our people leave us feeling this way. Every job has it's bad days. Every person has an off day. BUT it should absolutely not be a regular thing and should definitely not be the norm.

Now that we have a list, what can we do about this? Obviously, we can't just cut every person out of our life and we can't just up and quit our jobs immediately. I mean, that sounds awesome, but it's not really realistic in most cases. So what can be done today?

Well, let's start with the toxic people in our life. First, make a promise to yourself that you will distance yourself as much as appropriate (depending on your situation of course) from the toxic people you know. Some people will be easier to distance yourself from and some people will be harder. Understandably, it's oftentimes difficult to distance yourself from family, coworkers, etc. So just start small. Maybe start with people that you are not required to see on a regular basis. Maybe just promise yourself that you will say no to invitations from people that you feel are toxic.

Here's a pro tip: one quick way to start building your self-esteem is to keep your promises to yourself. Seriously! We talked earlier about the importance of not abandoning yourself but it's definitely worth mentioning again.

If you consistently put your feelings aside and cater to the feelings of others (including the toxic people in your life), you are essentially betraying yourself and that right there is one big bad vibe! So, start with baby steps and let's start distancing ourselves from bad vibes. If you are hating your job and it's bringing you down, what can be done to change that? Is there anything about your job that could change and make it better? Could you talk to your boss and try to make some improvements? If not, how about working on putting together a new resume? Maybe start thinking of different career options? Just start brainstorming. What do you envision when you see yourself going to your dream job? What type of feelings do you envision feeling? What qualities would make a job perfect for you?

Goodbye guilt! When distancing ourselves from toxic people and situations, it can oftentimes cause major guilty feelings. In my past I have had to say sayonara to several soul suckers. And I always felt guilty. I always beat myself up over it. I always thought I needed to have a really valid reason for saying goodbye. But, here's the thing, you don't have to have any other reason than the fact that you don't feel good around them. That's it! You don't need any other big excuses. You don't need any "proof." You can literally just say to yourself, *you know, I always feel like crap around this person so see you later, alligator!* That's it! And, even better, you can feel good about it! You are literally sticking up for yourself and practicing self-love when you give the boot to toxic people. So, no need to feel guilty! Pat yourself on the back and kick the guilt to the curb. Plus, earlier we talked about the danger of carrying around negative feelings such as guilt. So, seems to me that it's time to kiss guilt goodbye.

Phew. We have done a LOT of work in this chapter. But, I promise you, it's all an important part of the process. I don't want you to skip out on any of this. When you really do the internal work and start incorporating these tactics into your life, the real magic starts to happen.

So, again I ask, what's weighing you down?

Chapter 7: *Loving You*

Alright, go ahead and buckle up, buttercup, because this is probably going to be the hardest chapter of this book for some. It's definitely the hardest for me. Why? Because we are getting on the self-love train. Oh yeah. No joke. So put your seat belt on and enjoy the ride because this ENTIRE book is a big old waste of time unless we can master this chapter. So, let's get this party started.

Let me start by saying that I have literally wasted so much time on this beautiful Earth hating myself. I have spent an embarrassing amount of time beating myself up for being me. I have spent years shaming myself for how I look, how I act, and how I breathe. But mostly for how I look. Yep, not kidding.

I have never been a teeny tiny person. I have never been one of those people with tiny little limbs that look like twigs that you could easily snap. I have never been one of those people whose hip bones are protruding when I stand up straight. I certainly have never been accused of being bony. Even at my skinniest, I still had a look of being athletic or sturdy. Eww, not sure I like the word sturdy.

When I was a kid, I was average. I never really had any kind of substantial weight problem until later in life. However, I was ALWAYS, as long as I can remember, battling with my body size. I was constantly consumed with believing I was fat and ugly. I remember feeling so ugly and so fat during certain times and events. Now, when I look back at pictures from those times and events, I am literally amazed at how I actually looked. My body was small! I looked fabulous!! I would give anything to go back to that little, cute figure I had.

But, at the time, I hated myself. I was convinced I was the most horrendous being on Earth and that I was the size of a humpback whale.

Today, when I stand in front of a mirror, I don't think, *oh my, you are one smokin' hottie!* But, I also don't think to myself, *oh my, you really should be banished from Earth for being so unattractive.* I have learned that, in the end, hating on myself doesn't help anything. I mean, what's the point? If anything, it makes EVERYTHING worse. It makes me depressed. It makes me want to binge. It makes me want to hide in my house for all of eternity. It brings my vibe down to zero. And that's a real problem!

Since one of the main points of this book is to do away with all that makes us feel bad (or at least 95% of it), then hating ourselves has got to go. It's pointless and it just makes everything worse. And, in my opinion, it keeps us from ever really having the body of our dreams. You know the body I am talking about? It's the beautiful, healthy, trim body in which we feel good in our clothes and feel confident walking into a party in. It's the body that we are not starving ourselves for or shaming ourselves into. It's the body that is nourished properly with good food and good love. That's what we are shooting for! And you can't beat yourself up to get this body.

Have you ever heard of manifestation? I am guessing you have. Well, one of the main, most important principles of manifestation is that your thoughts create your reality. What does that mean? Well, to sum it up, it basically means that if you sit around all day telling yourself that you are a fat, ugly, whale, subsequently, in a cruel twist of fate, you will be a fat, ugly, whale. Ouch.

This theory applies to every aspect of life. Your thoughts and beliefs shape your reality. So, if you spend your time thinking and believing that you are unlikeable, then that's the vibe you are giving off. And, guess what? People probably won't like you. Ouch again.

Sounds rough but, actually, knowing this is super exciting! Why? Because manifestation works for the good also! If you think and believe that you are a cutie, then that's the vibe you are putting out and, you guessed it, people will, most likely, see you as a cutie.

Remember how we talked earlier about the importance of what we are telling our bodies? Well, once again, you can see how dangerous it can be to talk to yourself in a negative way.

Something exciting that I have seen is the idea that you can manifest the body that you desire by thinking and feeling good thoughts about your body. For example, if you start actively working to think positive thoughts about your body and you start envisioning yourself living in your dream body, then you are telling the cells in your body to get on board the dream-body train and start bringing this vision to life! If you close your eyes for a few minutes a day and picture yourself in your dream body and really FEEL what it would feel like, then you are on your way to having this body in reality. But…you have to ditch the negative self-talk.

Let's consider manifestation by looking at the following two scenarios. What kind of outcome do you think these ways of thinking might produce? For these scenarios, let's pretend you are going to your high school reunion. I know, scary, right? But stick with me. Okay, this is you walking into the reunion:

Scenario #1: *Holy cow, I literally am a cow. I am standing here at this stupid class reunion and I don't even know why I came. Everyone else looks SO good and I am literally the ugliest person here. I look like a whale! I didn't do my hair right. My outfit is completely wrong. I hate myself so much. Why do I do this? Why do I let myself come to these events knowing that I am so ugly? I should be ashamed of myself. I have to get out of here. I am leaving and I am definitely going through the donut drive-through on the way home. Ugh.*

Scenario #2: Oh, I really don't love these reunions. But, I'm glad I came. I got to say hi to Stacy and I haven't seen her in years! And it's so crazy to see all these people after all this time! But I am getting tired and really want to make an exit. So I am going to say my goodbyes and head home because I REALLY want to take a bubble bath and get in my bed and read. Maybe I'll have a good snack too because I am really hungry. And I can't wait to get these uncomfortable shoes off!

Okay, so the difference here is pretty obvious. The events of the two scenarios are basically the same but the thought processes in each are completely different.

What kinds of outcomes do you think these scenarios would produce? For scenario #1, does this person sound like she is likely to be living in a healthy, trim, happy body anytime soon? Also, does she sound like a very approachable, appealing person? My answer to both of those questions would sadly be no.

Now look at scenario #2. Does this person sound like she is in a good headspace to create a healthy, trim, happy body? Probably so. Also, doesn't she sound much more approachable and attractive to you?

Which scenario would you rather be in? Which scenario do you think is healthier to your well-being and mindset? Let's say that, in each scenario, your body is exactly the same and your outfit is the same and your hair is the same. Essentially, every single thing in the two scenarios is the same except for your mindset and your thoughts. If you had to choose either scenario to live through, which would you choose? I am guessing that you would choose scenario #2. I am guessing that you would choose to not be focused on thinking about hating yourself. I am guessing that you would choose to not live in misery. I am guessing that you would choose to be free from beating yourself up. So, let's work on choosing that NOW!

I know, I know. It's really freaking hard to change your thoughts and start easing up on yourself. But, when you really take a good look at the two scenarios above, you will see how blatantly pointless the negative thoughts were in scenario #1. I mean, what good did they do? What purpose did they serve? How did they help?

Okay, I can hear you now. You are probably saying, "well, those negative thoughts fueled me to kick my butt into gear and lose the darn weight!" Well, maybe so. But also, maybe not. More likely, they fueled you to punish yourself through starvation. Either way, my point here is, do you want to live your life in a constant state of hating yourself or would you like to live your life free from the obsessive thoughts of misery?

Let's say that you're told that you will 100% definitely lose the exact amount of weight you want to lose over the course of exactly two years. Would you rather spend the next two years beating yourself up and hating yourself and living with miserable thoughts? Or would you rather ditch the bad thoughts, try to think good thoughts, and just try to enjoy the journey? I personally would choose option #2. In a pinch, I would rather think good thoughts and maybe be a little happier along the way.

I also am a big believer that if you can't be happy now with the way things are then you won't be happy either when you get the things you want. I mean, maybe for a hot five seconds you'll be happy. But, if you haven't given negative thinking the old heave-ho and trained your mind to let that shit go, then you probably will be no different in the future.

Think about people who win the lottery. Apparently, the majority of winners blow through their winnings within just a couple of years. The majority of winners find themselves right back in their previous circumstances. Why? Because they didn't change their mindset. In their minds, they were still broke. In their minds, they were still lacking. In their minds, they were still unworthy. So, unfortunately, they manifested themselves right back into their former living conditions. Oof.

Think about it this way. If you continue to diet, you are letting the universe know that you are overweight and need to diet. Therefore, you will just keep on attracting more pounds and more dieting into your life. On the other hand, if you ditch dieting and trust yourself to eat healthily, you are letting the universe know that you've got this. You are letting the universe know that the weight is coming off and you no longer need to diet. This is why our mindset and how we talk to and treat ourselves is so darn important.

Have you ever heard the phrase, "fake it until you make it"? I am guessing that you have. Well, I am bringing it up here because I want us to start incorporating this into our daily lives. This is how we are going to put manifestation into practice and start living like people without any weight issues. Sound good?

Let's start by envisioning two women. One of the women is heavyset and the other is thin. Picture them both standing right in front of you. Okay, got it?

Now let's take out a piece of paper and make two columns. One column is for the heavyset woman and the other is for the thin woman. In each column we are going to write down a thorough list of thoughts, feelings, and actions that we imagine each woman might have.

Here's an example of two lists I came up with. After reading these, you may be able to expand even more and that's awesome. Just write down everything you can think of.

Take a look a look at these two lists.

Heavyset woman:

1. I have to constantly watch what I eat.
2. I can't go swimming because I will look too fat in my bathing suit.
3. I have to count every calorie.
4. I am ashamed of myself.
5. I am unlovable.
6. I need to hide my eating.
7. I hate how I look.
8. I can't ever cheat on my diet.
9. I can't be trusted around food.
10. I can't go to the gym until I lose twenty more pounds.
11. I am too embarrassed to take a walk in my neighborhood because I am so out of shape.
12. I can't apply for my dream job until I have lost the weight.
13. I can't lose the weight.
14. I don't think I will ever be happy with my body.
15. I can't put myself on the dating website until I lose the weight.
16. I can't buy those cute clothes until I lose the weight.
17. I am not worthy of being friends with people who are thin.
18. I am not comfortable around thin people because I am so fat.

Thin woman:

1. I don't let the shape of my body hold me back from doing anything I want.
2. I can go swimming without being overly concerned with how I look.
3. I love to eat healthy, nourishing food and I also love splurging from time to time.
4. I make choices based on what feels right to me and not how I look.
5. I go for walks in my neighborhood and go to the gym without feeling embarrassed by my body.
6. I am worthy of being friends with people of all shapes and sizes.
7. I don't need to hide anything I eat.
8. I can trust myself with food.
9. I don't really put a lot of thought into what I eat and I definitely don't obsess over food. It's just food.
10. I deserve to be loved for the person I am.
11. I love my body for what it is and I love taking care of it.
12. I am concerned with my health and how I feel more than the number on the scale.
13. If I want to eat a piece of cake, I eat a piece of cake. I don't stress over it or beat myself up afterwards. I don't overthink it.
14. I don't check my weight every day and I don't really think about my weight much.

Okay, can you see and feel the difference between these two lists? I am hoping that you have come up with even more examples that could be added to these lists. Why is this stuff important? Well, let's dive in.

I am going to ask you to start playing the role of the thin woman. I want you to make a complete list of the things you think a thin woman would say, feel, and do and then I want you to start saying, feeling, and doing those things! I want you to pretend you are an actress playing the role of a thin woman! Well, maybe that sounds a little bananas but I am hoping you catch my drift.

What's this about, anyway? Well, like I mentioned before, you can start to manifest the body of your dreams when you start to embody the thoughts, feelings, and actions of a person with that body. When you start thinking, feeling, and acting like a thin person, you are letting the universe know that you are becoming a thin person! I know, this may be pushing the limits of woo-woo for some people, but I really believe in it!

Here's the thing. I don't believe that you can successfully achieve becoming a thin, happy, healthy person while you are still embodying the characteristics listed in the "heavyset woman" column. I just don't believe that's possible. I mean, yes, technically you can become thin while having those characteristics. But will you be happy and healthy? I don't think so. I don't know about you but I also want to be happy and healthy! Thin is not my only goal.

So, let's do this. Let's start embracing the thoughts, feelings, and actions on the "thin girl" column and see where that takes us. Go ahead and go swimming. Go ahead and buy the cute outfit. Go ahead and apply for that job. Go ahead and be happy. You will be officially putting the universe on notice that you are becoming a thin, happy, healthy girl! And the universe will have no other choice than to get on board with this plan. How cool is that?

Okay, so we have seen how manifestation and our mindset works. Now let's dive into the good stuff. It's time to figure out how we can start loving ourselves. I know this may seem like an uphill battle but we can do it. We have to. We have to start treating ourselves better. We have to start loving ourselves and treating ourselves with compassion. We have to give ourselves some grace. I know, you are probably thinking, *okay great, sounds wonderful, but how on Earth do we do that??* Well, I have a magic trick for this. Read on.

Do you have a daughter? If not, do you have a niece or some other young, female family member? If you don't have any of these, just picture a little girl. Maybe a little girl around seven or so years old. Okay, I want you to close your eyes and picture her. Picture her standing in front of you. Picture her a few pounds overweight. You could maybe consider her a little chubby (I hate that word, but I am trying to get you to envision this little girl in a certain way). Really get a good vision of her. See her standing there and think of how young, impressionable, and vulnerable she is. Think of how innocent she is. Maybe she is holding her favorite doll. Maybe she is sucking her thumb. You see her and you just want to scoop her up and give her all the hugs. She is so sweet and adorable.

Now picture her turning and looking into a mirror. She gazes at herself in the mirror and says out loud, "You are so ugly. What a stupid, fat, ugly, little girl you are. Why can't you control yourself? You are worthless. I am ashamed of you! Why do you continue to fail? Why can't you just be normal like everyone else? Why can't you just stop eating! You don't deserve to ever be loved."

Please hand me the tissues because, I don't know about you, but this breaks my heart. Thinking about this gets me every damn time. When I think of my daughter (or any young girl), ever talking to herself this way, I just cringe. I stop in my tracks and feel appalled. I want to shake her and say, "do you even see how beautiful you are?? Do you even see how valuable and worthy and adorable you are? Do you even see how your smile lights up the whole room? Can you even comprehend how very much you are loved?" I would have so much compassion, love, and grace to offer her. I would want to hold her in my lap and hug her and tell her everything was going to be okay. Don't you agree?

So, for the love of humanity, why don't we extend this same grace to ourselves? Why don't we show ourselves the same outpouring of love and compassion? Why don't we see our own inherent value that has absolutely nothing to do with the numbers on the scale? Why don't we see how beautiful we are? Why don't we see how cruel we can be to ourselves?

When I look in the mirror, I should be saying to myself, *girl, your body is fighting this fight! It is getting you through this life and hasn't given up on you yet! What an amazing thing. You may not yet be where you want to be physically, but every damn day you get yourself out of bed and try again and that makes you one bad mother trucker!* YES!!! Amen to that!

Right now, I want you to start addressing the little girl inside of you. I want you to start picturing the five-year-old version of you when you talk to yourself. Or maybe picture a little miniature version of yourself tucked into your shirt pocket listening to everything you think and say. How will you start speaking to yourself now? Can you see yourself showing your body a little more compassion?

For instance, let's say you've had a nightmare of a day and you trip up and eat a gazillion cookies. How will you now talk to the little girl inside of you who just had an awful day? Here is what I tell myself now when this kind of thing happens. "Girl, you had a CRAP day. You did your best to avoid the cookies but today that just wasn't happening. NO. BIG. DEAL. It's seriously okay. Enjoy the damn cookies and tomorrow you can get right back on track. I love you."

Wowzas. What a difference! In the long run, do you see how tremendously powerful this can be? This kind of talk takes away the need for any punishment and instantly breaks the never-ending binge/starve cycle. How? Well, you have just eliminated the starve. And, when you start talking to yourself like this more frequently, I promise you that you are also going to do a lot less binging.

So, what else can we do to stop hating ourselves? Here's a few ideas.

Listen to yourself. Listen to your thoughts. Catch yourself when you are in a shame spiral. Just notice the self-hatred thoughts and acknowledge them. Most of the time our minds are on autopilot and we don't even notice we are hating on ourselves. So, just try to consciously make an effort to notice when you are thinking bad thoughts about yourself. Write them down when they happen if you want. You will be absolutely amazed at how often these thoughts can happen and how horrible they sound.

Another trick is to stop in your tracks and acknowledge these thoughts. Sometimes just acknowledging them and actually seeing what you are doing is enough to stop it. I mean, when you really stop, acknowledge it, and see how silly and useless these thoughts are, it's easy to just think, *nope, not today, thank you. Good vibes only for me please.* Or, when you stop and acknowledge that you are in a shame spiral, take a few deep breaths and think to yourself, *okay negative thoughts, I hear you trying to weigh me down but you're really not helpful and you're only bringing me down. So you can get going now.*

Another trick that I have heard is helpful to some is to counter the negative thoughts with good ones. So, when you catch yourself hating on yourself, stop and acknowledge first. Then, force yourself to think of five positive things you like about yourself. Or five positive thoughts about your body right now. This might look something like this:

Okay mind, I hear you thinking all this negative nonsense, so here's what I think.
#1: I may be a few pounds overweight, but I am still an awesome human.
#2: I am waking up and trying my best literally every day.
#3: If I slip up or have a bad day, that just means I am human. And, let's face it, people who never slip up and never have bad days are just not normal.
#4: Somebody, somewhere, would give anything to have the life and the body that I have.
#5: I literally woke up this morning healthy and breathing with another chance at living my best life and that is freaking amazing!

Okay, the last thing I want you to do is learn how to catch yourself in a negative spiral and reverse it by giving yourself a pep talk. I want you to become your own best cheerleader. I want you to practice this like it's a government mission that you have been assigned to complete. Really! It's that big of a deal!

You can do this pep talk, like we did before, envisioning your young self if you want. However you choose to do it is fine. But the kicker here is that you have to do it looking in the mirror. Yikes! I know. But this is non-negotiable. Sorry!

You have to look in the mirror and speak these words to yourself. You can write them out ahead of time if you want. The only recommendation I have is that you really give this some thought and carefully choose what you want to say. The words need to be powerful to you. They need to be able to pull you out of a funk. They need to be strong enough to reverse a bad mood. They need to leave you feeling like a boss when you are done. Get it?

I'll go first. Here's mine:

Okay girl, listen here. I hear you hating on yourself and you are just wrong. You are literally beautiful! I see you getting out of bed every morning and giving it your all and I just couldn't be more proud of you. You have been through so damn much and you are still smiling, showing up, and busting your ass and that is freaking amazing!!

And if you could only see how absolutely beautiful you are through the eyes of others, you would be amazed. I am serious. You have a heart of gold. Please, please, please don't waste your precious time or energy thinking bad things about yourself. You don't deserve it. I wish you could see how amazing other people think you are. I can't even begin to tell you how much I love you. You mean everything to me.

What do you think? I'll be honest. This can feel level-ten bonkers at first. But after some time, it gets easier and starts to be really impactful. After getting used to it, it's now hard for me to look in the mirror and speak these words without getting a little tearful. But that's the point. I want you to speak such love to yourself that you are instantly softened. You drop the cold, hard negativity and sink into warm, loving, compassion. Sounds good, doesn't it?

I promise you that if you start incorporating some of these tactics, you will start to find some compassion for yourself. You just might even start to love yourself! So, break out that mirror, ditch the negativity, and start loving on that little girl inside of you. She deserves it.

Chapter 8: *But Why?*

Over the years I have embarked on multiple diets for multiple reasons. I have gone on an immediate crash diet after receiving an invitation to a summer party that would involve a cute little cocktail dress. I have purchased New Year's Day diet programs that promised to have me looking good in a bikini by summer. I have been to the doctor and been mortified by the number on the scale and immediately started a diet involving only eating zero-calorie food so that, when my next appointment came around in twelve months, I would beam with pride when I stepped onto the scale and made my doctor proud. And I have tried desperately to lose the pounds before going to Disneyworld so that I didn't feel too fat to fit on the rides and I didn't embarrass my kids.

Now those all seem like very valid reasons to buckle down and drop the pounds. But they never worked. Oh, I may have lost a few pounds from time to time. But it always crept back.

Here's the thing. When I finally reached a point where I quit wanting to lose the weight for external purposes, that's exactly when the freaking weight started coming off!! Like magic!!

Somewhere along the line, after years and years and more years, I literally became exhausted from even thinking about trying to please other people. I just didn't care so much anymore. And it was not at all that I was depressed or giving up on life. It was the opposite! I was actually, drumroll please, starting to care about myself! I know, CRAZY.

I was starting to care more about my health and my feelings and my comfort levels than about how Joe Blow at the cocktail party thought I looked in my summer dress. Oh, let's be honest, I definitely was still self-conscious about my looks and of course I still wanted to look good in my jeans, but my attitude was shifting more towards pleasing myself than pleasing others.

I started thinking things like, *I don't want to feel physically uncomfortable anymore or like I am squeezing myself into this freaking chair. I don't want to get diabetes and die. If I don't feel like an absolute goddess in that darn cocktail dress, then I am just not going to the party and that's that and I couldn't care less. I would rather stay home and read a book in my pajamas anyway!* I literally just stopped caring (for the most part) about what other people thought. I started putting myself first and caring about my body, my health, my comfort, my LIFE!

Here's an example of what I mean. For the longest time, I wanted to lose weight, buy some new cute outfits, and get my friends to set me up with a certain single guy. I envisioned myself looking sooooo good in my new body and my new clothes and, in my vision, I was the happiest me ever. I would be looking so good, dressed in my new perfect outfit, getting ready for my first date in years. I would be a little nervous but feeling so good about my cute new shape and how I looked. The doorbell would ring and I would open the door and there would be Prince Charming at my doorstep. And I would feel so confident and pretty and put together. And Prince Charming would fall madly in love with me.

Well, that hasn't happened (yet!). But here's the thing. For years I held this vision in my head of this scenario. And, in order to make it come true, I put giant heaps of pressure on myself to lose weight. I starved myself. I beat myself up. I compared myself to other women. I berated myself for not looking as good as other women who I assumed that, because they had pretty figures, must have perfect lives and be living in a constant state of happiness. I chose pleasing a random guy that I had never met over pleasing myself. Ugh. I starved myself, beat myself up, and put my body through the ringer to win the (possible) affections of a person that didn't even know me. What on Earth?

At some point along the way, I realized what I was doing. I realized that my "why" was all screwed up. I realized that I would never truly lose the weight or be happy if I was doing it for anyone else and not solely for ME.

And, I will be honest with you, this can be a hard habit to kick. To this day, if you mention to me that there is a party coming up or you know a cute single guy, my first thought might be, *okay what diet can I start tomorrow to lose the most amount of weight in the quickest amount of time.* Yuck.

All this people pleasing and caring what others think and trying to impress others just became exhausting. I just grew weary of being stuck in this cycle and it became glaringly obvious to me that it wasn't working. Obviously, the pressure I put on myself to lose the weight before the big event was not working. And, quite frankly, it was most likely contributing to the problem. And the starvation diets and beating myself up for the imaginary guy weren't really getting me anywhere. They were, most definitely, making matters worse.

So, this is the point in time when my reasons for losing weight became more about ME and less about anyone or anything else. This is when I decided to consciously start trying to please myself before anyone else. This is when I said to myself, *screw literally everyone else, I am looking out for me now.* And the damn weight started coming off.

No joke. As soon as I shifted my mindset from pleasing others to actually caring about me and my body, that's precisely when losing weight became easier.

But let me stop right here and say that this, most likely, isn't something that can be faked. You have to actually get to the point where you truly care more about yourself and your health than impressing others or just looking good in a bikini. If you are not feeling comfortable yet in that cocktail dress, you have to be willing to say, "you know what, I am going to skip that damn cocktail party tonight because I am not feeling like I look super hot and I am going to, instead, choose to stay home and take a bubble bath and watch a good movie and read that good book and take care of myself and my feelings. I am not going to submit myself to feeling shame or self-loathing. I care too much about me for that kind of nonsense." Of course, if you are feeling the love for yourself and you just know that you look so good in that cute little dress, then, by all means, go to the darn party!! Go on and have an incredible night and live it up!

My point here is that you have to reach a point where you are making choices and doing things that make YOU comfortable. You are doing things that feel good to YOU. You are choosing yourself first and you absolutely refuse to put your sweet self into a position that will make you feel bad. You are choosing YOU.

This can absolutely, 100% be done without being "selfish." And if someone thinks you are being "selfish" for putting your comfort first before going to a cocktail party, then you may want to rethink that person's vibes anyway. If you have a friend that makes fun of you for wanting to eat healthy or wanting to take up cycling, then it may be time to show them the door anyway. You may have been, all along, doing hurtful things to yourself just to please this person.

I had a friend who, when I was around her, I always felt pressure to eat crap. And if I said no or acted like that wasn't what I wanted to do, she would make it sound like something was wrong with me. I guess misery really does love company. I had to get myself to the point where I was truly okay with turning down offers to hang out with her. I had to be okay with letting her go. I had to mentally get to the point where my comfort and my health and my needs were no longer something that could be sacrificed to please her. And, since I am a lifelong people pleaser (eww), this was a really hard thing to do.

I think this can be summed up by presenting two different scenarios and looking at the impact each could potentially have on your well-being, health, and self-esteem.

Scenario #1: *Ugh, I am dreading going to this cocktail party. I haven't lost the weight and I am so fat and ugly. I have two weeks until the party so I am going to have to starve myself and eat only boiled eggs until then because, if I start now, maybe I can lose 15 pounds before the darn party. It would literally be soul crushing for anyone to see me looking the way I am now. Honestly, I don't even want to go to the party but I have to go because, if I don't, my friends will be mad at me and then I will feel like crap for pissing them off and they may quit inviting me or they may make a big deal about it.*

Scenario #2: *Oh yeah, that cocktail party is coming up soon. Okay, well I will wait and see how I feel about it when it gets here and make a choice about it then. If I am feeling confident and party-ish that night, then I will go. And if I am feeling self-conscious and not party-ish that night, then I won't go. End of story. Whether I go to the party or not will be determined by me and my feelings and NOT by the feelings or thoughts of others. My decision is about taking care of myself and protecting my mental health and not about appeasing others. I will be sure not to commit myself ahead of time to being someone's ride home or someone's designated driver so that, in case I decide not to go, I haven't messed up someone else's plans.*

Do you see how different these two thought processes are? In the first scenario I was willing to beat myself up and torture myself to win the approval of others. In the second scenario, I did my best to not mess up anyone else's plans, but, at the same time, I put my self-care first.

After realizing that my "why" was all wacky and backwards, I made a decision to put myself first. In doing this, I had to decide what people I could still give away my energy to without losing my complete focus on making a radical shift in self-care. The only two people I decided on were my two kids. After thinking about it, I realized that my kids were the only two people on Earth who I would sacrifice little bits of myself and my energy for. Everyone else was an adult and could fend for themselves.

Maybe you are thinking this sounds really harsh? I know, it does. But, the thing is, in order to shift my mindset and change my life for the better, I had to, for the first time ever, reserve all of my energy (minus my energy I give to my kids) for myself. I had to take a stand for myself and say to myself that I am important. I am deserving of my time and energy just as much as my friends and my coworkers and my job and my everything else. I had to stop sacrificing my needs for the needs of others.

So, I decided that, aside from my kids (and I am a single mom so I don't have a husband, otherwise I would have included him), I was putting myself first. No more going to lunch with a friend when I really wanted to go to the gym and workout. No more helping out with work on the weekends when I really wanted to spend the days doing yard work and writing. No more going to a dreadful party when I would rather stay home and watch a movie.

Of course, there will always be things you are obligated to do and can't get out of. Or there will sometimes be an instance where a friend or work really need you. But those aren't the times I am talking about.

And, here's the thing, if your "why" is based on other people or events, there's a solid chance it won't pan out anyway. You may not run into that cute guy at the concert after all. You may get a terrible stomach bug and have to miss the class reunion anyway. Or you may lose the weight and run into the super cute guy at the party but he still isn't in to you anyway. Ouch.

Anyway, it was during this time that my "why" started to shift to healthy, helpful, loving reasons. I started to see things differently and I wanted to lose the weight for different reasons. I stopped being willing to starve myself to impress another person. I stopped being willing to eat the cake just to make someone else comfortable. I got my mind right.

Here are some of my "whys," in no particular order:

1. I don't want to get diabetes.
2. I don't want to feel bloated or physically uncomfortable anymore.
3. I want to feel light, flexible, and like I can run up a flight of stairs if I need to.
4. I don't want to feel tired all the time.
5. I want to walk into a clothing store and be able to fit into most clothes on the rack.
6. I want to be able to cross my legs comfortably.
7. I want to feel comfortable in airplane seats.
8. I don't want to be sickly as an older adult.
9. I want to be vibrant and healthy until I reach an old age.
10. I want to be able to run and play on the playground with my future grandkids.

11. I want to have good mental clarity.
12. I no longer want to be depressed about how I look.
13. I don't want to waste another precious minute on Earth feeling bad.
14. I don't want to struggle with bending over to tie my shoes.
15. I don't want to have trouble physically getting out of bed in the morning.
16. I don't want achy joints.
17. I want to feel healthy, fit, and active.
18. I no longer want to feel held back by my weight.
19. I no longer want to feel the pain of being overweight.

Okay, first, let's sit down and take a good, honest look at what your current "whys" are. And be really honest! Are you trying to lose those last twenty pounds because you know you may run into that guy at that party next month? Are you trying to drop a quick ten because you know you might have your picture taken in that work photo they are publishing on Facebook next week? Are you starving yourself before the class reunion?

While there is nothing inherently wrong with these tactics, we want to get ourselves to the point where our "why" shifts to a more health-centered, long-term approach.

After writing down our current "whys," let's take a look at them. Are there any on your list that seem focused on pleasing someone other than you? Are there any that seem like they are focused on a purely superficial reason? Are there any that focus on a one-time event? If so, let's see if we can acknowledge these as being about pleasing someone else. Let's see if we can understand that these "whys" may be more about the needs of others and less about our own health and happiness.

Now, let's start making or adding to our list of "whys" that are more about our own health, own comfort, and our own happiness. Well, and maybe also about the health, comfort, and happiness of our children and/or immediate family as well. I mean, if you want to lose the weight to walk your daughter down the aisle in her wedding, that's a pretty valid "why." But, if you want to lose the weight because you may possibly run into Joe Blow at a concert next month, we are going to need to add some more "whys" here.

Now that we have some "whys" listed, let's start working on making these "whys" the first priority. If you feel yourself having the urge to starve yourself because you just heard that guy someone told you about is going to that party next week, maybe take a few deep breaths and gently remind yourself that you are looking out for you and you are in this for the long haul and starving yourself is maybe not the best plan. Or, if you are at the shoe store and you find the absolute cutest pair of shoes and you go to try them on and notice that it's really freaking hard to bend over, maybe make note of this as a good "why" for your list.

Once you start finding your own "whys," it can start to feel super empowering. Just remember, the most important aspect of any "why" is that it is centered in focusing on you and your best interests. It does not focus on pleasing others. When you can really get this concept nailed down, you will be in the sweet spot for weight loss.

So why do you want to get healthy and lose weight? Why do you want to live out the rest of your life in your best body? Why do you want to put yourself first and nurture, respect, and love your body?

Why?

Chapter 9: *Feeling Good*

Alright, let's keep this train moving. Next up? A ride on the feel-good express. I know, I'm a weirdo. But it's currently like 5 AM and I am probably a little loopy. Or, more likely, this is just normal me. Whatever.

Anyway, this chapter is all about finding ways to bring more "feel-good" vibes into our lives. Who doesn't want that? Remember how we talked earlier about manifestation? Well, here it is again.

When we feel good, we attract more people, experiences, and things into our lives that feel good. It's like, if you are vibing in the feel-good atmosphere, you will be like a giant magnet attracting more things that feel good. And, equally so, if you are vibing down in dumptown, it's going to be more down-in-the-dumps type stuff that comes your way. No, thank you.

I believe that when we start feeling good about our lives, we enter into the perfect mindset for letting go of excess weight. I believe that, when we truly start learning to feel good, we no longer need to carry around the baggage. So, let's start looking at some ways to feel good.

What am I even talking about when I say feel good? Well, no, I don't just mean physically feel good like having no aches and pains. I mean, that's great, but what I am really talking about is mentally feeling good. Sometimes it actually takes some practice and intentionality to feel good. It is so super easy to get stuck in a rut of feeling one way or the other. It is so super easy to get stuck in a certain vibe.

Have you ever seen those movies where there's a character who seems like a curmudgeon and then this person comes along and pushes them out of their comfort zone a bit and then they start changing? They start laughing, having fun, and feeling happy? Well, this is what I am talking about. Sometimes we need a little push or a change in how we do things to start feeling good. And the exciting thing is that sometimes even the smallest changes can get us headed in the right direction.

In the town where I live, there is a gym that I have been going to since I was in high school. It's just a regular gym or "athletic club" or whatever you call it. The front entrance to this particular gym is a high-ceilinged, large entryway with a check-in desk. Nothing super extraordinary. But what I want to mention here is the way that I feel when I walk through those doors.

Every time I enter those gym doors, I immediately feel my blood pressure drop and my shoulders loosen. I feel a sense of calm wash over me. Why? Well, the entryway has a waterfall wall so there is the sound of falling water in the background. Also, there is always the perfect amount of essential oil scent floating in the air. And the décor gives the vibe of earthiness and health and well-being. I feel like I am in a spa. I feel suddenly grounded and centered. I feel GOOD!

On days when I've got my act together, I often infuse essential oils or melt scented wax or light candles in my house. I am big on things that smell good. After a long day at work, when I am coming home exhausted and spent, walking in my back door to a spa-scented house instantly lifts my spirits and makes me feel so good. I feel my blood pressure lower and my muscles relax.

Now that I have figured out that good smelling things make me feel good, sometimes when I am frustrated, or furious, or tied up in knots with anxiety, I will go in my bathroom and open one of my scented oil bottles and inhale deeply. It doesn't always make me feel like a Buddhist monk in meditation, but it definitely relaxes me some. I would imagine that the combination of the good smelling oil and my deep breathing are the perfect mix for calming my nerves.

And speaking of deep breathing. Deep breathing has become like my best friend. It works! At some point along the way, I realized that, when I really thought about it, I wasn't really breathing ever. I mean, obviously I was breathing. But I mean, I wasn't really BREATHING.

I started this weird thing where, every once in a while, I would try to "catch myself" breathing. Like, out of the blue, I would stop and check in on how I was breathing. Well, nine times out of ten I found that I wasn't really breathing. My breathing was usually shallow and seemed ineffective. So, I would intentionally take a few deep, calming breaths. And it is absolutely amazing what a difference that makes. It really does make you feel better. I mean, after running around for years and doing nothing but shallow breathing, slowing down and taking some good, deep breaths feels really good! It's like you can feel your body oxygenating. You can feel your cells doing their little oxygen happy dance. Yea, that's really weird, but you get it. Anyway, you can add deep breathing to my list of things that make me feel good.

And, little side note here, there are starting to be lots of "breathwork" classes and courses popping up that seem really cool. And guess what? Several of them incorporate weight loss into the intended results. From what I have seen, there is lots of evidence that breathwork is a legit tool to help your body live her best life. Anyway, a quick Google search would probably lead you to some info.

What's next for feeling good? One thing that works like a charm every time for lifting my spirits is taking a drive. What? I know, maybe that's weird. I got it from my Dad. In my family, when you've just been cooped up in your house for too long or, frankly, when you are home and can't think of anything better to do, you take a drive! To no particular place. For no particular amount of time. For no particular reason. We just get in the car and drive. Preferably alone. But, unless we are driving each other nuts at the moment, family or whoever can come along. The point is to just get out of the house and get some air and see some sights and listen to some good music. Or maybe listen to that audiobook or podcast you are currently obsessed with. Whatever. No real rules to this. It just seems to work wonders for me.

So, what are some things that get you feeling good? What are some things you can do on a daily basis without much effort that instantly lift your spirits? I mean, of course jetting to the Caribbean or going for a day-long spa retreat will probably get you feeling pretty good, but what can you incorporate into your everyday life without expending a ton of effort or a ton of money? What are some little things that just make you feel good and cozy inside?

The point of this chapter is for you to start considering what makes you feel good and start doing more of it! This is going to help you raise your vibe and keep it higher. This is going to get you feeling good! And, remember, when you feel good, you are in the right mindset or "vibe" for successful weight loss. And, I mean, who doesn't want to feel good anyway?

Here I am going to list some of the things that have been proven to make me feel good. I am listing these just to give you an idea of what I am talking about here and to help you get started brainstorming. Then I am going to get you to make your own list. So, here we go:

1. Anything that smells good. Preferably, spa-like smells. But, honestly, I am also a lover of the smell of burning leaves. And the smell of a campfire gives me all the feels.
2. Deep breathing. If I notice I am stressing, I will make every effort to stop for a minute and take several really slow, deep breaths.
3. Going outside. I love being outside. So, if I am at home and feeling anxious, I will just walk outside. Maybe pretend like I am checking the mail. Or maybe just walk around the

yard and pretend like I am inspecting the grass. Whatever. Just get myself outside.

4. Going for a drive. Good music. Good podcast or audiobook. Or maybe silence. No destination. No particular place to be. Maybe the windows down. Maybe the windows up. Sounds like Heaven to me.

5. Listening to music I love. Nothing calms me down more than listening to *Hallelujah* by Leonard Cohen. Nothing makes me feel more at peace than listening to *Let it Be* by The Beatles. I've got a whole list of songs that get me feeling good. I highly recommend making a playlist of favorite songs that instantly melt you into a peaceful, warm, comforted feeling.

6. Shopping in a store I love. There are a few stores in the area where I live that I just love going into and browsing. I don't even have to buy anything. Just walking in the door and smelling the scented candles, and looking at the pretty clothes, and listening to the soft background music make me feel good. There's one home décor store in my town that, after a good thirty minutes

of browsing, I feel like I just took a Xanax.

Okay, so are you getting the gist of this? We are purposefully seeking out things that make us feel good. And we are doing more of them! I have shown you some small things you can do so now let's look at some bigger things you can do.

Several years ago, I found myself in a complete funk. I was working the same old jobs, punching in and punching out. I was going home every afternoon and going through the same old motions. Wash the dishes. Do some cleaning. Take a nap. Still feel exhausted. Pay some bills. Cook dinner. Etc. Etc. Etc. On occasion, I would do something fun like going to a movie with a friend but, really, that was about it. I felt tired all the time. I didn't want to get out of bed in the morning. My eating and my pants sizes were equally expanding. I didn't feel very good about anything. This went on for a couple of years.

One day, out of the blue, a friend and I decided to start our own business. My aunt had sent me an email telling me about this new, cool type of business idea and it sounded like something right up my alley. I called my friend and told her about it and we decided to give it a try. We made a plan to have lunch the next week and start planning it.

It was at this exact moment that something in me clicked. I immediately felt an excitement inside myself that I hadn't felt in years. I felt hopeful and excited and I was looking forward to every day spent working on this. My friend and I started meeting for lunch every week or so and brainstorming and making plans and researching. For the first time in YEARS, I started springing out of bed in the morning with happiness. I was actually looking forward to the day! I hadn't felt like that in forever and I kept thinking to myself, *How could I have been living without this feeling for so long? This is exactly what's been missing from my life! It's like magic!*

Aside from the obvious value of feeling excited and happy, there was another benefit to this newfound magic in my life. All of a sudden, I wasn't really so hungry anymore! I mean, yes, I still ate and I probably still had my binge-type moments, but they were fewer and farther between. And, due to the fact that I could see a bright future ahead now, I instinctively had the urge to eat healthier. Without trying I suddenly wanted to look and feel better for my new business. I hadn't felt this way in a very long time. As a result, I started slowly losing some weight without even really trying! I just felt so good inside and it felt like being a heavy person just didn't go along with this new exciting life I was building.

Well, after several months of really trying to get our business off the ground, it just didn't work. And I felt really down again. What would make me spring out of bed in the morning now? What would I have to look forward to and get excited about? I felt pretty down for a bit of time and then, when I got sick of feeling that way, I made it a point to work my hardest to find something else to get excited about. Another project that made me want to get out of bed in the morning. Another source of magic.

So, take a look around and tell me what you see. Do you see magic? Do you spring out of bed most mornings of the week? Do you get excited about what your day ahead holds? Do you look forward to things you are working on?

If you don't see any magic, let's get you some! What can you do to bring some magic into your life? Do you have a hobby you always wanted to put time into? Do you have a business idea that you have been stuffing down for years out of fear? Have you always wanted to take that skydiving class? Whatever it is, why not do it right now?

Finding some magic in life has become an obsession of mine. Yes, clearly I have a tendency towards obsession. But, whatever. Anyway, from my own experiences in the past, I have found that, when I don't have much excitement going on in my life, food becomes my joy. I find that the only thing I have to look forward to when I go home from a long day of work at my mediocre job is what I will be having for dinner. My thrills come from the sugar rush I get from cake pops. Yikes.

Obviously, cake pop thrills are not the ideal source of excitement. So what else can we do to make our lives a little more magic? What else can you do to start filling the hunger inside of you? Get it?

It seems to me that, when our lives seem a little boring or we feel stuck in a rut, we are most likely hungry for more. And I don't mean food. Hungry for what then? Passion. Magic. Excitement. Purpose. Whatever makes you spring out of bed in the morning and look forward to the day.

It makes perfect sense to me that, when our "cups" are full, we no longer need to stuff ourselves with food. When we are living a life in which we feel fulfilled, happy, and excited, we are no longer hungry for more.

One last thing to mention. I believe that, when we find something to be passionate about, it helps to serve as a distraction from our weight woes. It takes the focus off our unhappiness with our bodies. How is this helpful? Well, aside from giving us a bit of a reprieve from our angst, it also stops our negative thinking pattern which we have learned is so detrimental.

Remember the importance of our state of mind being positive and manifestation? Well, again, if we are focused on how fat and unhappy we are, unfortunately, we are going to attract more fat and more unhappiness. When we switch gears and focus on excitement, happiness, and fulfillment, then, you guessed it, we get more excitement, happiness, and fulfillment. And that can very easily manifest in the form of a healthy, happy body. Sounds like magic to me.

So, let's get to thinking really hard of ways in which you can start to fill your cup. How can you find more passion and pleasure in your life? What can you do to start feeling more excitement? Maybe you can start thinking about taking that French class you always wanted to take. Or maybe you could start thinking about how you can start that small business. Or maybe you can head to the craft store and get the stuff needed to start that quilt you always wanted to make. Or sign up for that marathon and lace your shoes up.

One particular way to really get the good vibes flowing is to find something to do that, in some way, helps others. They say that the best feelings come from serving others. Could you maybe volunteer at the homeless shelter? Or go buy a few canned food items and drop them off at the food bank? Or maybe start sewing blankets for the hospital babies? Or even start writing a blog about your weight loss journey? You never know who might be reading and need to hear exactly what you have to say!

What are you going to work on today to get yourself vibing high? I promise that it will help you get in the groove for dropping the pounds. And, besides, who doesn't want to feel good anyway?

Chapter 10: *Check it Out*

Picture for one second that you are at the starting line of a marathon. You've been training for months. You've got the perfect running shoes. You've been eating all the right foods and getting good sleep. You've planned every step of this race in your mind for your whole life! So, you step up to the starting line, wait for the gun to go off, and start running.

But wait, there's something attached to your ankle, and it won't let go. You look down and there's a weight attached to your ankle, and it won't come off! You have to run the entire race with this godforsaken thing around your ankle! Twenty-six miles to go while being dragged down by this thing! How on Earth??

Well, you are still able to finish the race but, with this ankle thingy, it was way harder and much more frustrating. And you didn't break that world record like you were hoping to. Ugh!

What in the heck am I talking about and what does this have to do with anything at all? Well, my suggestion to you is that, if you have any type of underlying and, possibly, not yet known medical condition, you may be running an unnecessarily harder race. You may be dragging something around your ankle without even knowing it.

For multiple years after getting divorced, I felt like crap. Seriously. Physically, mentally, and spiritually I was drained, exhausted, and achy. I attributed it to stress and my diet and being overweight. While I am sure that stress and my diet probably were huge factors, what I didn't know is that my hormones were, to quote my doctor, "whackadoodle."

Somewhere along the line, after years of feeling miserable, fat, and defeated, I went to the doctor. I instantly fell in love with this doctor. I told her that I had been trying to lose weight, I had been feeling exhausted for years, and I had been through multiple stressful events. And she listened to me! She ran all kinds of blood tests.

Two weeks later I went back to see her to follow up about the lab work. As it turns out, I had been running my race with a weight tied around my ankle. My progesterone and estrogen levels were low, and my cortisol levels were off. So my doctor prescribed some supplements. And guess what, within a week or so, I started feeling better! I didn't change hardly anything about my diet, but with the supplements, I felt more energetic and clear headed. Amazing!

So, no, unfortunately my doctor did not have a magic pill to help me lose weight. Ugh. BUT, with the supplements she did give me, I felt better overall and this, in turn, made losing weight feel slightly easier. I had more energy, my mood was better, and I didn't feel exhausted and ravenous constantly like I had in the past. I felt like I was no longer dragging the ankle weight!

My point here is that, just make sure you are not being held back by some medical issue that you don't even know about. It will make things so much harder than they need to be. From what I have learned through my own experience, even the slightest little tweak in something like your hormones can have a big impact on your energy levels, mood, and overall feeling of wellbeing.

Let me stop right here and say that, in all honesty, for years I avoided going to the doctor and even mentioning that I didn't feel good. I didn't want to be a whiner and I was sure that the doctor would probably take one look at me and think, *This fat girl needs to get her stuff together and lose some weight and quit whining.* I felt certain that, if blood work was run, the results would come in and the doctor would inform me that, indeed, everything was normal and that I was just lazy and needed to stop stuffing myself. And there was NO WAY that I could survive hearing THAT. I beat myself up enough about being overweight. I certainly didn't need anyone else doing it too.

Anyway, my point in this chapter is that it might behoove you to just see where things stand inside your body. You may have absolutely no issues and that's really good news! But, you may have a few little things that need some tweaking and you will feel a little bit better.

Like I said before, in an unfortunate turn of events, my doctor didn't have a magic weight loss pill. Sigh. But she did get me feeling a little bit better overall and that just made my whole life a little easier. I didn't feel as exhausted, and I didn't need as many gallons of caffeine. I didn't feel as depressed and anxious and need as many donuts. I didn't feel as lethargic and want to sleep instead of going for a walk.

Do you have a doctor that you like and trust? Have you been in for a checkup recently? Do you know what's up with your insides?

Firstly, do you even have a physician or primary care provider that you jive with? Do you have someone that listens to you and makes you feel heard? Do you have someone that fits in line with your medical and healing beliefs?

If not, sit down and take a minute to figure out what kind of person you are regarding health and medicine. Do you prefer supplements (when possible) over medication? Do you like a doctor that has a good bedside manner or are you okay with someone being less "friendly" as long as they are board certified? Do you have a preference about male or female? Do you prefer someone with a clinic close to your house? Or are you okay with driving a ways to see someone you really like?

There are so many variables to consider. But I would imagine that you have some general idea of what your personal preferences are. So, make a list of them now.

Once you have your preferences figured out, start asking around. Ask friends, or people in your Facebook groups, or coworkers, or whoever. Start getting an idea of what your options are and pick a person that sounds fitting. And then:

1. Make an appointment!

2. Go to the appointment!

You may go to the doctor and be told everything is fine and dandy and you just need to lose some weight. Please don't feel bad about that. I had this happen to me and it REALLY sucked.

Here's what happened. A few years before going to my current doctor, I went to see my gynecologist for a routine appointment. I guess, at that point, my hormones weren't completely bonkers yet. But I was overweight. The doctor ran routine bloodwork and said everything looked perfect and I needed to "take off some pounds." Ouch. Even though I was fully aware that I needed to lose weight, having someone else say it (especially a doctor) felt horrifying. I was humiliated and beat myself up about it for days. I went into a serious shame spiral. And I wanted to eat cake for days.

Eventually, I pulled myself together and got over it. I realized that, yes, doctors do need to tell patients when it's time to lose some weight or else it may lead to health problems. Even though it kind of sucks to hear it.

So let's get those appointments made and get everything checked out just to be on the safe side. No dragging leg weights around here.

Chapter 11: *The Food and the Moves*

Y ou did it! You made it to the last chapter! Whoop, whoop! Okay, sit back down because we need to get through this last chapter to complete the process. In this section, we are going to discuss food and exercise.

I intentionally have left the food for the very last chapter because I so strongly believe that weight loss is not really about the food. I mean, yes, obviously it's about the food. But I believe it's much more about everything that we have talked about in the previous chapters. If you truly want to be successful in losing weight, I urge you to focus on the previous chapters.

It's, honestly, really hard for me to even discuss the food part because I have such mixed feelings about suggesting any particular way of eating. I am a believer that diet and exercise need to be tailored to every individual. I don't believe that there is a one size fits all diet or exercise program that everyone can follow and be successful with. I think there are some general rules that everyone can follow (such as avoiding existing only on cupcakes). However, I also think that every individual needs to look at what works for their own body. For instance, nuts may be wonderful for me, but they may cause a deadly allergic reaction in you. Yikes.

Anyway, I am going to tell you my diet and exercise story and explain to you what has worked for me. You can take it or leave it. You can tweak it to fit your own needs. You can read this and decide that I am bananas and go eat a pizza. It's all good.

I want to start by saying that I am sharing this way of eating with you because, in all my MANY years of dieting, this has been the one game changer. This has been my food miracle. And, like I said a gazillion times before, you really should run this past your doctor before you start. So, assuming all is good and you have the okay of your doc, let's get started.

A while back I was taking part in this self-improvement seminar. Yes, I LOVE all things self-help. I know, I'm bananas. Anyway, this seminar was a Tony Robbins event. FYI, Tony Robbins is one of my favorites and I highly recommend anything he does. Okay, sorry, back to the story. So, this seminar was four days long and involved all aspects of life improvement. The focus of the event was building a life you love.

Okay, so what does this have to do with food? Well, on the last day of the seminar there was this very brief talk given about diet and healthy eating. The portion of the talk that discussed food was literally maybe two hours. Which, in a four-day event, two hours is pretty tiny.

Anyway, during this talk the speaker mentioned the benefits of eating a plant-based diet. A what? I had only vaguely heard of eating plant-based before and had never really given it any thought. But, for some reason, this short little two-hour segment was one of the things that stuck with me the most out of the entire seminar. The speaker discussed the potential benefits of eating a diet consisting of mainly plants. He mentioned some studies that had been done which seemed to show undeniable health benefits related to this way of eating. I was intrigued.

After the seminar ended, I headed to Google and searched for info on eating a plant-based diet. At this point I wasn't even completely sure what this meant. Turns out that a plant-based diet is, for lack of a better word, a "cleaner" version of a vegan diet.

Okay, pump the breaks. If you are anything like me, you are thinking to yourself, *vegan? Like don't eat anything but berries and hug trees all day kind of vegan? Like exist on nothing but lettuce and live in a tent in the forest kind of vegan? Huh?* I know, I get it. This is exactly what I was thinking. Red flags were flying everywhere for me. The vision I had in my mind of "vegans" was not a vision in which I could see myself. Honestly, I was pretty sure vegans came from a different planet. But I am asking you to hear me out.

So, I did some research and found out that a lot of people are now referring to the vegan way of eating as "whole food plant-based." Or WFPB. Essentially, it's a way of eating that includes all vegetables, all fruits, nuts and seeds, legumes, and whole grains. No dairy and no meat. No animal products of any kind. Okay, before you run for the hills, just know that this way of eating DOES include potatoes and pasta. Just saying.

Anyway, after watching some documentaries about the benefits of this way of eating (no worries, I will provide links a bit later) and doing some googling, I decided to give it a try.

I want to start by mentioning that it was around this time that I had hit the highest weight of my life. Except for when I was nine months pregnant with my kids. Yikes. This time I was not pregnant. Just 100% fat. Ouch. Needless to say, I was willing to try just about anything.

One of my first realizations about the WFPB way of eating is that it is kind of weird in that, unlike any other way of eating I have ever encountered, as you may have already been aware, people follow this diet for not only health benefits but also for their beliefs about animal cruelty and environmental reasons.

So, I am going to be 100% honest here. I really love animals. I am pretty smitten with the Earth. But that is not why I chose to eat this way. I chose it for the purported health benefits. I chose it for the weight loss benefits. Of course I love cows and I think our Earth is definitely a keeper but that's not my number one driver for why I do this. I hope that doesn't make me sound selfish and horrible. But I am trying to be completely transparent and let you know that you can choose to eat this way for LOTS of reasons. You can choose it for the animals. You can choose it for the forests. You can also choose it for your waistline. You can choose it for ALL of these reasons.

Veganism, I have also come to find, can be political. I guess when you are talking about environmental issues and such, people have different ideas about the best way of going about things. That's totally fine. But getting political is not my jam so I stay away from that aspect of this way of eating. That's not why I choose to eat this way. I am just here for the rice and beans.

Anyway, back to my story, I did my research and decided that this was something I wanted to try. Why not? I had tried everything else. I may as well give this a shot. I also realized that, after finding out more about this way of eating, it seemed to resonate more with what naturally felt healthy to me. This way of eating included apples and bananas and that just felt right to me.

First, to give you some perspective, when I started eating this way, I was a full-blown eater of meat, dairy, and everything else. My typical day included eggs and yogurt for breakfast, tuna salad for lunch, and salmon and veggies (probably with some cheese somewhere) for dinner. And, of course, donuts and cookies on occasion. It was rare for me to have a meal without meat or dairy. So, this diet was no small adjustment for me.

I started out by completely cutting out dairy. No cheese. No yogurt. No butter. No milk that came from an animal. I had been drinking almond milk for a long time before this, so I didn't have to change anything about that. If you do drink dairy milk, just switch to a plant-based milk such as almond, coconut, or oat milk. Just no dairy.

I gave myself about a week or two of eating no dairy before I moved on to any other changes. But let me just say that giving up dairy can be HARD. The cheese cravings can be off the charts. Did you know that cheese is addictive? Really! It contains compounds that cause your body to release feel good chemicals and (obviously!) you are going to want to keep coming back for more of that! Anyway, it's a hard thing to give up.

Again, after this chapter I am going to post links and a list of a bunch of good resources for finding out more about all this stuff. Don't be thinking that your work is done with this book! I will briefly mention here that, after just a week without dairy, I had already dropped a pound or two. I had changed nothing else about my diet except for cutting out dairy.

Okay, so after a week or so with no dairy, I embarked on the train to no meat land. I went cold turkey and cut out all meat/animal products.

Now, this is the point at which I am going to need to start addressing the multitude of questions that I know you must have right now. Where will you get your protein? Don't you need meat to survive? What about iron? Aren't you going to be eating way too many carbs? Wait, what about tacos? Are you CRAZY? I know, I know. These are all the questions that I asked.

After doing an exhausting amount of googling and documentary watching, it turns out that, believe it or not, plants (veggies, beans, nuts, whole grains, etc.) have enough protein for us to do just fine on. Also, there are a gazillion awesome plant-based protein shakes on the market that taste yummy and have plenty of protein. I drink a plant-based protein shake almost every night. It's my "dessert." Unless I cave and have some cookies. Oof.

Meat. I thought it was going to be a LOT harder to give up meat than it actually was. Come to find out, it was harder for me to give up dairy. Someone at some point told me that when you are craving meat you might just be craving the items that oftentimes go along with it. For instance, are you really craving the hamburger or are you possibly just craving the warm bun, melted cheese, mayo, pickles, and ketchup? Well, turns out, I miss the mayo and cheese more than the actual meat itself.

One more thing I have heard mentioned several times about eating meat is going to be something that is considered just a few steps beyond crazy town for some of you. Yes, it sounds a little woo-woo but for some reason it really stuck with me. And, okay, I can be a little woo-woo sometimes.

Anyway, some people say that, when we eat animals, we are ingesting not only their tissues but also all their emotions and feelings that are stored in their tissues. Huh? Well, remember earlier how we talked about "the issues are in the tissues" like Mastin Kipp said? I assume that this is what's going on here. I don't know about you but, like I said just a minute ago, the last thing this girl needs is MORE emotions or feelings. Especially if they are negative. No thanks to feeling like a caged animal. Anyway, this is a pretty out-there concept and you can, of course, take it or leave it. I just thought I would mention it in case it resonates with anyone else.

For me, personally, ditching the meat was more of a mental game than anything. It was hard, at first, to feel like I wasn't harming myself by not eating meat. I was concerned about the protein. It just didn't seem normal to not eat meat. I mean, what in the world would I eat on Thanksgiving Day? No turkey? But, in time, I started getting comfortable with it and now I don't even think about meat much anymore. I know, so crazy.

Carbs. Oh holy carbs. Carbs and I have been in a love-hate relationship for my entire life. For at least the last ten years I have been actively struggling to avoid them. They have been like a drug to me. The sugar. The bread. The yumminess. And considering that the most recent popular diets have been along the lines of keto, Atkins, and carnivore, it's REALLY hard to switch gears and look at carbs in any other light besides being the devil. But, and I know this may seem impossible to some, I am going to ask you to make carbs your friends again. I know, I know. CRAZY. Let me explain.

I have spent the better part of my adulthood avoiding carbs at all costs. You want me to eat that chocolate cake? I can't! I will gain ninety pounds! You want me to eat a banana? Are you a PSYCHOPATH?

The thing is, for as long as I can remember, I have spent ungodly amounts of energy avoiding carbs but, at the same time, craving them like there's no tomorrow. I succumbed myself to a tortuous, ongoing battle. Every single time, in the end, carbs were the winner. I would avoid them for days and then fall off the wagon and stuff myself with all the bread. I would count each individual carb and declare victory when I stayed in the single digits. But then, inevitably, I would cave to my cravings and devour triple digits of carbs in a single sitting. Yikes.

What's crazy to me is that, all the while, I kept thinking to myself, *I just don't understand how apples are "bad" for you. I can't grasp the concept of choosing cheese over grapes just because the cheese has fewer carbs. Aren't apples grown in the Earth? Didn't Mother Nature intend for us the eat these fruits and vegetables from the Earth?* In my mind, avoiding nature's fruits and vegetables just didn't seem right to me. It didn't make sense in my brain that these could be the foods that we should avoid. I was internally confused about how bacon could be considered healthier than fresh papaya. Anyhow, I put aside my questions and continued to avoid carbs because that's what the current diet trend said to do.

Well, cut to the first few weeks of me following a plant-based diet. I had to rewire my brain completely to even consider eating an apple. A bowl of oatmeal? You must be kidding. I grappled for at least a few months with whether or not I was harming myself and making matters worse by eating carbs.

But, here's the thing, when you cut out meat and dairy, you have to add in foods with carbs or else you really will be stuck eating just lettuce. Also, there is actually lots of evidence that your body really does do best when you are eating healthy carbs such as fruit, whole grains, and starchy vegetables. Who knew?

So, here's what happened. I slowly convinced myself that it was okay to start eating healthy carbs again. I started eating fruits, oatmeal, potatoes, rice, starchy vegetables, etc. And, honestly, it felt like Heaven. I felt satisfied again! I would eat a meal and walk away feeling like I wasn't missing anything!

And, here's the best news yet. Are you ready? Drumroll, please...I LOST WEIGHT!!! Yep, not lying. The pounds started, slowly but surely, falling off. I wasn't hungry. I wasn't counting calories. I wasn't counting carbs. I wasn't intermittent fasting. I wasn't doing anything besides eating whole, healthy, plant-based foods. As much as I wanted.

Within just a few months I had lost eighteen pounds. NO JOKE. I am not even kidding when I say that this felt like the pigs were flying, the sea had parted, and Mother Theresa had risen from the dead. A gosh darn miracle. When you have been battling the scale for YEARS and losing and gaining back the same five pounds over and over, losing eighteen pounds without really trying feels like you just reached the top of Mount Everest. Amazing.

Okay, let's recap. Here's what I was eating. Fruit (all kinds), vegetables (all kinds), oatmeal, brown rice, quinoa, nuts, seeds, beans (all of them), and any other nutritious, yummy, plant-based foods. On occasion, I also ate pasta, cereal, bread. But not frequently.

Let me give you a few examples of my typical meals and then I am going to go a little deeper with some tips and tricks.

Typical breakfast (as much as I want):
Oatmeal with berries and flaxseed OR
Fruit and rice cakes with peanut butter OR
Salad- kale, spinach, veggies, granola, dressing

Typical lunch (as much as I want):
Salad-kale/spinach, veggies, dressing OR
Spring rolls with Thai peanut dressing OR
Veggies with rice and beans OR
Veggies and avocado sandwich OR
Veggie sushi OR
Hummus wrap

Typical dinner (as much as I want):
Veggie sushi OR
Veggies with rice and beans OR
Veggie burger and fries OR
Veggie lasagna OR
Sweet Potato and veggies OR
Lentil soup and salad

Typical snacks (as many as I want):
Fruit OR
Rice cakes/crackers with peanut butter OR
Plant based protein shakes OR
Veggies and hummus OR
Peanut butter and jelly sandwich

Okay, before you look at this list and run for the hills, please know that, if I can do this, anyone can. Literally. Also, please note that this list does not include occasional chips, occasional cookies, occasional French fries. And this list, by no means, encompasses all the foods I eat. This is just a small sample. To give you a better idea of some of my most frequently eaten meals, I am going to put a few recipes at the end of this chapter.

The only strict rule I follow is no meat and no dairy. I also try my hardest to eat minimal added sugar and minimal or no oil. Other than that, I try to eat as clean as possible within the confines of a vegan diet. I say this because it's technically possible to eat a really unhealthy vegan diet. After all, Oreos and French fries are technically vegan. Really!

But I want to point out here that, since you will be consuming more carbs on this way of eating, there's a high probability that your cravings for carb-rich foods will decrease. I know mine did. It's hard to crave something sweet after you have had beans and rice and fruit. You tend to feel more satisfied on this way of eating. Hallelujah!

There are several tips and tricks I want to give you to make this easier. I also want to point out how to maximize your potential weight loss through focusing on calorie density and cutting out oil/fat.

I am not going to go deep into the scientific details, but I want to explain how focusing on calorie density works and why it can be so essential to weight loss.

As you probably already know, the different food groups (fats, starches, proteins) have different amounts of calories per gram. Carbohydrates have the fewest calories per gram. What does this mean? Well, this means that you can consume MORE of the foods that have a lower calorie density.

For example, one cup of popcorn has maybe thirty calories. One cup of avocado has about 230 calories. So, for weight loss purposes, you will want to eat a cup of popcorn instead of a cup of avocado. This does not at all mean that avocado is bad for you. It just means that it has a higher calorie density so you may want to consume smaller portions of it. Instead, focus on eating more of the low calorie density foods.

A good idea, at first, is to start paying attention to calorie counts (not counting calories!) so that you can get a general idea of which foods have higher calories per gram/serving. Focus on consuming more of the lower calorie dense foods. The nice thing about this way of eating is that by cutting out meat and dairy, you have automatically cut out most of the higher calorie dense foods.

Next you will want to watch out for consuming too much oil, too many nuts, or too much peanut butter, etc. When you consume lower calorie dense foods, it feels like you have to stuff yourself all day to get ENOUGH calories. Imagine that.

One trick I swear by and try to do as often as I can is to fill myself up first on lower calorie foods before I eat my "main course." For instance, I will have a giant salad or a bowl of vegetable soup before I have a plate of rice and beans or veggie lasagna. This way, I automatically eat a bit less of the more calorie dense foods.

I have also started eating salads for breakfast almost daily. This might be a bit out there for some people, but I swear it helps! Plus, it feels good knowing that you started your day with a big bowl of veggies.

I will take a minute here to talk about oil. Olive oil, coconut oil, canola oil. All of them. The thing is that they are pure fat and SO high in calories.

People have differing opinions on the health benefits of consuming oil. I don't know who's right and who's wrong but I do know that it has a gazillion calories.

I know, cutting out all oil probably sounds impossible. But I will say, I have managed to cut out almost all oil and I believe it's helped tremendously in my weight loss. I have also noticed a drop in my blood pressure and resting heart rate. I don't know if that's due to no oil or the WFPB way of eating in general but, either way, I'll take it! Anyhow, at the very least, I recommend reducing your oil intake.

Next up, sauces and dressings. Sauces and dressings have become my obsession. When you are trying to eat SO many veggies, it really helps to have a variety of super yummy sauces and dressings on hand. That way, even if you are eating the same types of veggies pretty frequently, you will feel like they are different because of the change up in flavors from the different sauces and dressings. There are several store-bought dressings that I am obsessed with but there are also a gazillion recipes for incredible tasting WFPB dressings and sauces. And, let me tell you, I pour that crap on everything. Just try to keep it low fat, low calorie, and vegan.

Let's take a minute to talk about fiber. There is so much evidence supporting the idea that fiber is of huge importance in our diets. It's also majorly lacking in keto-type diets. In the WFPB way of eating, you will get tons of the good stuff! Oatmeal, prunes, chia, beans, apples, broccoli, bananas, lentils, and more. Fiber for days. It will help you lose weight AND keep you regular. Yes!

Okay, I can imagine that you may be thinking, *this is all fine and dandy when I am cooking at home but what about eating out? What in the heck am I supposed to eat at a restaurant??*. Well, no worries, I have had no problem finding food on this journey. Believe me, I am a master at finding food. I regularly have to eat out because of travel and work. In my experience, there is ALWAYS something you can eat at almost any restaurant. It may not be ideal, but you can find something.

Again, this is a case where we want to try, if possible, to stick to the two main rules of no meat and no dairy. At most restaurants you can find pasta with marinara, veggies, baked potatoes, salads, rice, beans, etc. At fast-food restaurants, you might look for veggie subs/sandwiches, hummus wraps, salads, etc. Even Burger King has a vegan hamburger! I haven't tried it though so I can't give it a thumbs up or a thumbs down.

Recently, while traveling, I was in a small airport that did not have much of a food selection. The only restaurant was a fast-food place that had burgers, chicken sandwiches, and fries. Nothing else. Not even salads. Well, I was starving so a lunch of French fries and ketchup it was! And you know what? I had two large orders of fries with a mound of ketchup and I enjoyed every single finger-licking good bite. No regrets. I had no other choice for food so I figured I may as well go ahead and enjoy the darn fries! Of course, you don't want to have French fries and ketchup for lunch every day but sometimes is 100% okey dokey. Actually, lots of people these days are using air fryers to make French fries and those would totally be in line with WFPB eating. Yum!

By now you might be thinking, *okay, this is sounding like a LOT of vegetables! I mean, I normally eat eggs and bacon for breakfast. Now you want me to eat a dang salad? Are you nuts?* I know, I know. I seriously used to feel the same way.

Here's the exciting thing. Did you know that you can train your body to crave different things? Huh? Yes, really! There is more and more evidence coming out that shows that the gut has a little mind of its own and, depending on the type of bacteria it contains, you will crave different foods. Different foods produce different gut environments.

Why does this matter to you? Well, let's say you eat nothing but candy apples. Your gut will then be filled with candy apple loving bacteria. Subsequently, you will crave candy apples because your little gut bacteria are screaming, "more! more!". Alternatively, if you eat nothing but kale, your little gut bacteria will be the kind that love kale and will be causing you to crave more kale.

When you consistently eat healthy foods and do your best to minimize the not so healthy foods, your gut bacteria will accommodate and start wanting more of the healthy foods. Eventually you just might be craving salads for breakfast. I'm serious!

Okay, it's time to talk about the sweet stuff. Sugar. Sugar has been my enemy number one for as long as I can remember. Sugar has also been my best friend, comforter, and most reliable source of good feelings. Over the years, I have tried every possible trick in the world to beat my sugar habit. It has been an ongoing battle that I still struggle with. Ugh.

A while back I heard some unexpected but freeing information. I heard that it helps to treat sugar like any other drug. Treat it like heroin or cocaine. When you view it as a true addiction (which science shows that it truly is!), you may be more successful in kicking it.

When I started thinking of sugar as a drug, it shocked me to think of the willpower that's truly required of people wanting to give it up. I mean, sugar is EVERYWHERE. You'd be hard pressed to go to a party or restaurant without having it staring in your face. Now imagine if that was cocaine. Seriously! Think about how hard to resist it would be if you had a cocaine addiction and you went to a restaurant and there were different cocaine items on the menu. Or you went to a party and there was a buffet table set up with cocaine on nice little platters. Seems bananas doesn't it? Just think of that next time you go to a party and there are cupcakes and brownies set out. Makes you feel like you must be a superhero if you can resist that kind of temptation!

Another benefit of treating sugar like a real drug is that, at least for me, it amps up the seriousness of it. If you treat this like you have a real addiction (which science says you may!), you are more likely to find yourself making quitting a bit more of a priority. You may start thinking to yourself, *geez, this is kind of serious! I may need to give a little more effort to getting myself unhooked from this stuff.* For me, when I view it as an addiction, I start thinking things like, *okay, we have a crisis here. I am seriously going to have to drop everything and focus all my attention on fixing this. This is a true health crisis!* May sound dramatic but, honestly, it has helped me to ditch the stuff. So bring on the drama!

Anyway, we all know sugar is bad for our health. If you can manage to quit the stuff, I seriously recommend it. At the very least, try your darndest to keep it to a minimum. I know, it's HARD.

Speaking of addiction, what are you drinking? Another one of my biggest addictions has been diet soda. Nothing tastes better to me than an iced-cold diet soda. I don't know what is going on with these drinks, but they are seriously addictive. I have managed to give them up now but, let me tell you, it was a long trip on the struggle bus to quit. If you are anything like I was and you can't go a day without a diet soda or two, I urge you to give this habit up. More and more evidence keeps coming out about how bad for you this stuff really is. You will definitely be doing your body a huge favor if you can ditch the diet drinks.

While we are on the subject of foods that are hard to give up, I want to talk quickly about the idea of having "cheat meals" or "cheat days." I know some people strongly believe in them and some don't. I lean more towards the side that believes in them. But, first of all, I don't call them "cheat days" because that implies that you are on a diet. I call them "exhale" days.

From my own personal experience, I have found it helpful to, maybe once a week or so, have an indulgent meal that feels "forbidden." I feel like it mentally lets me release and have a moment of pure pleasure that feels so refreshing. I feel like I can "exhale."

Don't get me wrong, I feel like the foods I get to eat in the WFPB lifestyle are super delicious and filling. But, when I have a "exhale" meal, I allow myself to eat whatever the heck I want. Usually, it doesn't involve meat or dairy. But it, most assuredly, involves bread and sugar!

Another reason I like having "exhale" meals is that I feel like they create a more "normal" eating pattern. For instance, think about someone you know that has no extra weight and never diets. Most likely, they eat a relatively healthy diet but, occasionally, for birthday celebrations, while on vacation, or for whatever other reasons, they may splurge a little and treat themselves. They most likely feel no shame or concern about splurging because they know they will be right back to healthy eating the next day. They don't overthink it and definitely don't feel guilty about it. So, if you indulge in an occasional "exhale" meal, you are actually just copying a "normal" eating pattern like that of someone with no weight issues.

Anyway, you can decide what works best for you. I find that occasional "exhale" meals (or days!) feel like I am coming up from under the water for a deep breath. Once I have it, I can go back in the water and be just fine for quite some time. But if these meals throw you off completely, you can avoid them.

Alcohol. To be honest, I am not much of a drinker. Maybe two or three times a year, I will have drinks while out with friends. It's not because I am actively trying to avoid it. I just have no desire for it. I always seem to wind up with a hangover and nothing makes me more miserable than feeling nauseous. My "drug" of choice has always been sugar. You might relax with a martini. I relax with a cinnamon roll. Oof.

Anyway, I believe we each know our own bodies and can make the choices that seem appropriate for us. If you feel like alcohol is an issue for you, I would urge you to try to tackle it. If you feel like you can't go a few days without having a drink, then maybe there's something going on there. No shame in this. Just information. Regardless, I guess we can all agree that it's just extra calories.

Moving right along. Okay, I'm going to be honest with you here. There are like a million incredibly delicious WFPB recipes out there. A quick Google search or social media search will bring you a plethora of meal ideas. But, the truth is, I am no cook. And my kids would tell you that that's an understatement. Oof.

So, when it comes to eating this way, I pretty much eat the same things day in and day out. And the truth is that it gets boring. But you know what I have found? Getting bored with my food has turned out to be a blessing in disguise. I don't get super excited about eating anymore. Wait, what?? I know. Me, who is the queen of daydreaming about cookies, just said that I no longer get super pumped about my meals. I am more like, *oh, beans again? Okay. I'll eat later.* Now this might sound like the most impossible thing that you have ever heard. I know, right? But I am promising you that I am serious!

Here's the thing. If I put in a little effort and tried a bunch of the amazing looking WFPB recipes that are out there, I might not feel this way. I may never get bored with my meals, and I may look forward to every bite. If you have any kitchen skills, you may find yourself successful in cooking these recipes that turn out looking like a magazine ad. And that's great! That might get you all pumped about WFPB foods. It may make it easier for you to eat this way forever.

Or, if you are more like me, you might be lazy and put the same meals on repeat and lose oodles of weight because, shockingly, you can no longer muster up the excitement for another bowl of rice. Either way, seems like you will win! My point is, sometimes getting bored with your eating is actually okay.

By this point, you may be thinking, *but what about pizza? What about tacos? What about cheeseburgers??? You seriously want me to go the rest of my life without ever eating these again?* I know, I thought these exact same these. But, guess what? I have exciting news! There are now vegan versions of literally every food! Really! If you can get yourself to a Whole Foods or Trader Joe's or a similar grocery store, you will find oodles of vegan versions of all of the classics. And, no, they don't taste that bad!

For Mother's Day this year, my kids surprised me and made reservations at a vegan restaurant in the city near our home. We had chips and "queso." We had "chicken" nuggets. We even had tacos! And the greatest part is that it was actually yummy! I mean, yes, of course it tastes different and it takes a little getting used to. But it was good! And the more you eat this stuff, the more you like it. I now find myself occasionally craving the tofu "chicken" nuggets. Bananas! I used to think I would rather jump off a mountain than try tofu and now I crave the dang stuff. So crazy!

So, I have just thrown so much information at you. What are you thinking? You may be feeling like I haven't given you concise enough rules or parameters. Let me provide here a summary of the things I want you to consider focusing on.

1. No/minimal meat and no/minimal dairy.
2. Eat foods that are lower in calorie density.
3. Limit your intake of high fat foods such as oils, nuts, avocado.
4. Avoid added sugars.
5. Avoid processed foods/vegan "junk."
6. Eat ALL that you want of ALL vegetables, ALL fruits, ALL whole grains, ALL legumes.

Okay, got it? If you have social media, I am going to be listing some incredible social media accounts that you may want to follow. They share some amazing recipes and go into a little more detail about tweaking this way of eating for weight loss results. Plus, they are super inspiring and may help to get you pumped about eating this way.

I also want to mention here that I want you to make it a point to check in with your doctor if you decide to go full speed ahead with plant-based eating. Why? Because you may need to monitor your levels of some key vitamins and nutrients along the way. It's important to make sure your vitamin B12 levels are up to par. Lots of vegans supplement with vitamin B12 because you can only get vitamin B12 from animals or dirty vegetables that have just been pulled from the ground. Vitamin B12 comes from organisms in the dirt. Also, vegans usually supplement with a good plant-based Omega-3. Lastly, it's a good idea to monitor your iron and protein levels. I have a tendency to become anemic so I keep a close eye on these. But, not to worry, I had issues with anemia even before eating this way. Anyway, just make it a point to let your doctor know that you are eating this way and they will know what to look out for.

Last thing about the food. I just want to reiterate the importance of you doing what is right for your body. Going plant-based may not be in the cards for you. Maybe you will do better if you eat mostly plant-based and throw in a little meat here and there. Maybe this is not a way of eating that you are even remotely interested in. Okay, that's totally cool. Maybe focus your chosen diet on getting as many veggies as you can. Maybe there is some other reason that this way of eating may not be right for you. That's okay! I would just encourage you to still try to get lots of veggies and avoid sugar and processed foods. Also, you can always practice the calorie density trick no matter which way of eating you choose.

Honestly, I am still taking this day by day. Who knows what next year will bring? I can't guarantee that I will never eat meat again. I can't guarantee that I will never again succumb to the occasional cravings for warm queso. I can't guarantee much of anything. All I can say is that this feels good for today. And it has produced some pretty great results so far. Beyond today, who knows.

Okay, let's move on to our last topic. The moves. The exercise. Here's a bit about my story.

About ten years ago, on any given Saturday, you might find me at the starting line of a marathon.

No joke. I went through a phase of about six or seven years when I exercised like a freak of nature, and I participated in multiple marathons and triathlons. It makes me tired just thinking of it.

Anyway, this was a phase of my life in which I was a thinner person. But here's the thing. I ate whatever I wanted (including donuts, cake, pizza) but I POUNDED my body with tortuous workouts to prevent weight gain. I ran for miles and miles and then went home and ate donuts. I swam until I thought I might drown and then went home and devoured pizza. It couldn't have been "healthy." As much as I love the body I had during those years, I can't even imagine going back to those extreme exercise rituals.

These days I walk. Yep. I just walk. I take a nice, long walk almost every day. It lasts about 45 minutes to an hour. Out in the beautiful sunshine with my headphones in. Listening to some good music or an interesting podcast. I don't do a whole lot more in the way of formal exercise. I try to go to Pilates or yoga on occasion. I keep saying I am going to get back to doing some swimming. But, for now, I just do a lot of walking.

I will say though that I am a mover. I can't sit still for long periods. I get antsy and like to move around. When I am home, I move a lot around my house. I do laundry, dishes, general cleaning. I also cut the grass with a push mower. I move furniture around. I take the trash out. After I have been sitting for a while, I will get up from the couch and run up and down my stairs or hallway for just a couple of minutes.

The point is, I try to move a lot. And I try to do some of it outside. I am a huge fan of sunshine. Hello, vitamin D! I regularly can be found standing in my yard and soaking up the sun. I try to go outside at least once a day and soak up a few minutes of the warm rays. I highly recommend it!

Okay, so my only recommendation for exercise is going to be that you get some. Take a long walk. Go to a yoga class. Cut the grass with a push mower. Do some jumping jacks in your kitchen. Get in the pool with your kids and do some laps. Run up and down the stairs in your house. Whatever! Just try to move some every day.

Another quick point I want to make here is that my exercise (walking) has become just as much, if not more, about my mental health as it is about my physical health. There isn't much that a long walk in the sunshine with some good music can't cure. I believe SO strongly in the power of exercise to help with depression, anxiety, etc. It works wonders.

Phew. We have been through a LOT. Summary of this chapter? Eat plants and move around. The end. Seriously!

Chapter 12: *The End*

To wrap things up, let me tell you about the results I have had by doing everything we have talked about in this book. First of all, I have lost weight. Relatively easily. Without starvation. Without counting calories. With lots of carbs! I have lowered by blood pressure and resting heart rate. I no longer have the weird, bloated stomach that I used to have. My body no longer feels achy.

I have let go of a lot of old regrets and negative feelings. I have become more peaceful. My self-esteem is much higher. I have compassion, grace, and love for myself. I mean, I still have my days, but they are fewer and farther between.

Anyway, I no longer beat myself up. I stick up for me. I say no (or try my hardest to) when I mean no. I make time for me. I also push myself to get outside of my comfort zone. I make sure I take a walk most days of the week. I make sure to get some sunshine most days of the week. I take bubble baths and sometimes go get massages. I try to slow down and feel all my feelings so that I won't stuff them down later with ice cream and cookies. I meditate on most days. I pray a lot. And, since I am not now and never will be perfect, sometimes I eat the donuts.

I really hope this book has been useful to you. Really. I am a bleeding heart when it comes to weight loss struggles. I feel the PAIN. I feel sure that losing weight has been the biggest struggle of my life. And considering that my life has included losing both of my parents at younger ages, money struggles, divorce, foreclosure, almost bankruptcy, and being a single mom, I think that says a lot. Weight loss is HARD.

I want you to also remember that nobody is perfect. Nobody. And I would bet my money that you would be really hard pressed to find someone who has lost weight easily and without struggle. Why am I telling you this? I want you to remember that, even when you eat the donuts, you are still in the game. Even when you spend an entire day eating cookies, you are still headed in the right direction. Weight loss is never a straight and narrow course. There are bumps and setbacks along the way. And that's okay! They are part of the journey.

If you are anything like me, you have spent your entire existence wanting to lose the wait like yesterday. You want to drop the pounds as fast as possible and be done with it already. Well, I have come to the conclusion that weight loss really is a matter of "slow and steady wins the race." I am convinced that it takes real time to do the work to permanently change your mindset and transform your body in a non-traumatic way.

So, please give yourself time. Please be patient with yourself. Please remember how beautiful you really are and how precious your one-and-only body is. Please remember to be gentle with yourself and remind yourself every day that you are doing the very best you can. Because you are!

Like I said earlier, I just don't believe it's all about the food. It's about what's going on inside of us. It's about our pain. It's about our anger, fear, and hurts. It's about so much more than being hungry. But it's also very much about our hunger. Our hunger to be fulfilled. Our hunger to be free. Our hunger to be loved.

I wish you nothing but the best in your journey. I send you all the good vibes for finding the happiness you so deserve. I wish you health, happiness, and freedom. And I pray that you find peace with your body. You deserve it!

xoxo

Recipes

These are some of the staples of my diet. They are quick, easy, and don't require "fancy" or expensive ingredients. Remember, I have like zero skills in the kitchen, so you won't find anything complicated here.

Yummy veggies

This is the recipe for veggies that I eat almost every day. I typically use broccoli and cauliflower but you can use any vegetables. I usually eat some of the veggies fresh out of the oven and then freeze the rest in individual serving-sized containers. These are super easy to reheat in the microwave. I eat them as is or I top them with Salad Topping (recipe below) and dressing or sauce. Yum!

3 bags pre-washed, pre-cut vegetables
Mrs. Dash (or any no-salt seasoning mix)
Salt/pepper

Heat oven to 380. Line veggies on parchment paper-lined baking sheet. Sprinkle with Mrs. Dash and very small dash of salt and pepper. Bake for about 15 minutes.

Breakfast oatmeal

Oatmeal (steel cut, old fashioned, etc.)
Berries/bananas/any fruit
Ground flaxseed
Cinnamon
Water

Add water to oatmeal and heat to desired consistency in microwave. Top with fruit, flaxseed, and cinnamon. Enjoy!

Rice and beans

Quick cook brown rice (1bag or enough for 2-3 servings)
2 cans of beans (pinto, black, or any kind!)
Mrs. Dash
Salt/pepper

Cook rice following package instructions. Rinse beans. Heat beans in microwave or on stovetop. Mix beans into rice. Sprinkle with Mrs. Dash and pinch of salt and pepper. Again, I eat some when they are ready and then freeze the rest in individual sized containers. Perfect to reheat for a quick snack or meal!

Breakfast, lunch, or dinner salad!

You can really use any veggies for this salad but this recipe seems to be what I always go for.

3 cups chopped kale
2 cups baby spinach
½ cup diced carrots
½ cup Salad Topping (see recipe)
½ cup chickpea granola or other vegan granola
¼ cup low fat, low sugar dressing (I am obsessed with the Skinnygirl dressings!)
Mrs. Dash

Toss all ingredients in a giant bowl and enjoy!

Apple dessert

1 apple
Handful of raisins
3 prunes
1 ½ tablespoons peanut butter
Ground flaxseed
Cinnamon

Chop all fruit up into bite-sized pieces. Place in microwave-safe bowl. Heat about 2 minutes. Top with peanut butter, flaxseed, and cinnamon. Eat while warm. Reminds me of apple pie!

Dessert smoothie

There are so many possibilities when making smoothies! You can use ANY fruits, plant-based protein powders, plant milks, veggies/greens, nut butters, cocoa, cacao, flaxseed, hemp, chia, avocado, oats, and on and on and on!

2 whole frozen bananas
1 serving plant-based protein powder (any flavor)
½-1 cup of plant-based milk depending on desired consistency

Mix all ingredients in blender. Enjoy!

World's fastest lunch/snack

1 potato (sweet, russet, Yukon gold, any kind!)

Wash potato and trim about ½ inch off ends. Wrap in damp paper towel. Cook in microwave for 5 minutes. Voila! Sprinkle with cinnamon or salt and pepper or other seasoning if desired. I cook sweet potatoes all the time and throw them in my purse and eat them as a snack while I am out running errands or working. Seriously!

Quick rice cake snack

Rice cakes/crackers
Natural peanut butter
Raisins/prunes/other fruit
Ground flaxseed
Cinnamon

Add toppings to rice cakes and enjoy!

Salad Topping

This is a super yummy "topping" that I use in all different kinds of ways. I add it to salads. I add it to the Yummy Veggies recipe and call it lunch. I top sweet potatoes with it. You can do anything with it!

2 bags frozen corn
2 bags frozen soybeans
Mrs. Dash
Salt/Pepper

Heat oven to 400 degrees. Spread all ingredients on parchment-lined baking sheet. Sprinkle generously with Mrs. Dash. If desired, add dash of salt and pepper. Bake for approximately 15-20 minutes. Freezes great and is super easy to reheat!

Spring rolls

These are so yummy and super low in calories! And you can switch up the dipping sauces for different flavors. I have these for lunch or dinner several times a week.

4 rice paper spring roll wraps
Chopped kale
Shredded carrots
Alfalfa sprouts
Salad Topping (see recipe)
Dipping sauces

Prepare rice paper wraps following package instructions. Add ingredients. You can really use any ingredients that sound good to you! For the dipping sauces, I really like Thai peanut sauce and General Tso sauces. The brand, Sky Valley, makes some yummy ones. But you can use your imagination and come up with whatever you want!

Good Stuff:

This is a compilation of materials that I have found to be super helpful in my weight loss journey. Hopefully, you will find some of these to be helpful to you as well.

<u>Documentaries:</u>

Most can be found on Netflix, Amazon Prime Video or individual websites. Just Google search.

1. Forks Over Knives
2. The Game Changers
3. What the Health
4. Fat, Sick and Nearly Dead
5. Eating You Alive
6. Food Matters

Please note that there are a bunch of great documentaries on plant-based eating. If you want to explore further, just search the web.

Books:

This is a sampling of books that I have found invaluable in my weight loss journey. Some are about food. Some are about mindset.

1. The China Study by T. Colin Campbell, PhD and Thomas Campbell, MD
2. The Starch Solution by John McDougall, MD
3. Eat to Live by Joel Fuhrman, MD
4. The Secrets to Ultimate Weight Loss by Chef A.J.
5. Women, Food, and God by Geneen Roth
6. The McDougall Program for Maximum Weight Loss by John McDougall
7. The Body Keeps the Score by Bessel Van Der Kolk, MD
8. You Can Heal Your Life by Louise Hay
9. Finding Ultra by Rich Roll
10. The Blue Zones by Dan Buettner

Social Media Accounts:

Here are a few fun and informative Instagram and Facebook accounts.

1. @thebirdspapaya
2. @plantifulkiki
3. @highcarbhannah
4. @drnealbarnard
5. @oliviahertzog
6. @physicianscommittee
7. @dr.plantbased
8. @vegansvillage
9. @plantbasedonabudget
10. @thefeedfeed.vegan
11. @rabbitandwolves
12. @plantd.co
13. @medicalmedium
14. @nutrition_facts_org
15. @bestofvegan
16. @forksoverknives
17. @the.holistic.psychologist
18. @mastinkipp
19. @bluezones

Thank you so much for reading!

I hope you have enjoyed reading this as much as
have enjoyed writing it.
It would mean the world to me if you would leave a
review for my book! You can return to Amazon or
wherever you made the purchase and should be able
to easily leave a review.
Thank you so much!

You may also enjoy my other two books:
*The Three of Us: A Brutally Honest, Often Hilarious, and
Sometimes Heartbreaking Memoir of One Mom's
Adventures in Single Parenting*
and
The Single Mom's Little Guide to Building a Big Life

You can always keep in touch with me by following
me on Instagram and Facebook
@summerlinconner

Sign up for my newsletter to be the first to hear
about future books, courses, and other cool stuff!
www.summerlinconner.com

And, lastly, you can always email me at
summerlin@summerlinconner.com

I would love to hear from you!

Summerlin Conner is a mom, Registered Nurse, and author. When she's not spending time with her kids, Summerlin loves writing, laughing, and being outdoors. Summerlin and her kids live outside of New Orleans, Louisiana.

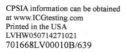